AN INTRODUCTION TO GENETIC EPIDEMIOLOGY

Edited by Lyle J. Palmer, Paul R. Burton and George Davey Smith

This edition published in Great Britain in 2011 by

The Policy Press
University of Bristol
Fourth Floor
Beacon House
Queen's Road
Bristol BS8 1QU
UK

t: +44 (0)117 331 4054
f: +44 (0)117 331 4093
e: tpp-info@bristol.ac.uk
www.policypress.co.uk

North American office:
The Policy Press
c/o International Specialized Books Services
920 NE 58th Avenue, Suite 300
Portland, OR 97213-3786, USA
t: +1 503 287 3093
f: +1 503 280 8832
e: info@isbs.com

British Library Cataloguing in Publication Data
A catalogue record for this book is available from the British Library.

Library of Congress Cataloging-in-Publication Data
A catalog record for this book has been requested.

ISBN 978 1 86134 897 5 paperback
ISBN 978 1 86134 898 2 hardcover

Cover design by Qube Design Associates, Bristol.
Front cover: image kindly supplied by Photodisc.
Printed and bound by CPI Group (UK) Ltd, Croydon, CR0 4YY

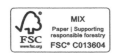

Contents

List of tables, figures and boxes

Tables

Figures

Boxes

Notes on contributors

Jennifer H. Barrett
Section of Epidemiology and Biostatistics, Leeds Institute of Molecular Medicine, University of Leeds, UK • j.h.barrett@leeds.ac.uk

Paul R. Burton
P^{3}G Consortium and Departmentsof Health Sciences and Genetics, University of Leicester, UK • paul.burton@le.ac.uk

Lon R. Cardon
Glaxo Smith Kline, Philadelphia, PA, USA • lon.cardon@gsk.com

David G. Clayton
JDRF/Wellcome Trust Diabetes and Inflammation Laboratory, University of Cambridge, UK • david.clayton@cimr.ca.ac.uk

Heather J. Cordell
Institute of Human Genetics, Newcastle University, UK • heather.cordell@newcastle.ac.uk

George Davey Smith
MRC CAiTE Centre, School of Social and Community Medicine, University of Bristol, UK • kz.davey-smith@bristol.ac.uk

Mylene Deschênes
Department of Social and Preventive Medicine and the Research Centre for Public Law, University of Montreal, Canada • mylene.deschenes@umontreal.ca

Shah Ebrahim
Department of Epidemiology & Population Health, London School of Hygiene & Tropical Medicine, UK • shah.ebrahim@lshtm.ac.uk

David M. Evans
MRC CAiTE Centre, School of Social and Community Medicine, University of Bristol, UK • dave.evans@bristol.ac.uk

Isabel Fortier
The P^{3}G Consortium and Department of Social and Preventive Medicine, University of Montreal, Canada • adesjar409@aol.com

Anna Hansell
Department of Epidemiology, Imperial College, London, UK • a.hansell@imperial.ac.uk

Andrew T. Hattersley
Wellcome Trust Centre for Human Genetics, University of Oxford, UK • andrew.hattersley@pms.ac.uk

John L. Hopper
Centre for Molecular, Environmental, Genetic and Analytic Epidemiology, University of Melbourne, Australia • j.hopper@unimelb.edu.au

Sarah Lewis
MRC CAiTE Centre, School of Social and Community Medicine, University of Bristol, UK • s.j.lewis@bristol.ac.uk

Mark I. McCarthy
Wellcome Trust Centre for Human Genetics and Oxford Centre for Diabetes, Endocrinology and Metabolism, University of Oxford, UK • mark.mccarthy@drl.ox.ac.uk

Lyle J. Palmer
Dalla Lana School of Public Health, University of Toronto, Canada • lyle.palmer@gmail.com

M. Dawn Teare
Mathematical Modelling and Genetic Epidemiology, University of Sheffield, UK • m.d.teare@sheffield.ac.uk

Nicholas J. Timpson
MRC CAiTE Centre, School of Social and Commu0nity Medicine, University of Bristol, UK • n.j.timpson@bristol.ac.uk

Martin D. Tobin
Departments of Health Sciences and Genetics, University of Leicester, UK • mt47@leicester.ac.uk

Acknowledgements

This book arose from a series on genetic epidemiology commissioned by the journal *The Lancet* in 2005. We are grateful to David Sharp at *The Lancet* for initially commissioning the series. The idea to turn the series into a book came from our observation that the *Lancet* series was widely used by academics in Europe and North America as a teaching aid or as the basis of short courses in genetic epidemiology, and our perception that the field needed a basic textbook in genetic epidemiology for a non-technical audience. This book has been written during an extraordinary time in human genetics; large sections of the original *Lancet* series written in 2005 are now wildly out of date after only several years – having been overtaken by the explosion of genome-wide association studies and the concomitant state change in our understanding of human genomics. This has introduced challenges of itself, and the book was deliberately delayed because of our wish to present a work that was as current and relevant as possible.

We are profoundly grateful to the staff of The Policy Press for their patience and good humour. We thank the authors for their diligent and timely revisions. We are very grateful to the loyal and hardworking members of the GenReach team in the Centre for Genetic Epidemiology and Biostatistics at the University of Western Australia – without the assistance of Anne Pratt, Ingrid Nilsson and Jess Lee this book simply would not exist. Finally, we each thank our long-suffering partners for tolerating the time spent away from family working on this book. We hope you like it.

INTRODUCTION

Lyle J. Palmer, Paul R. Burton, George Davey Smith

This book provides an overview of central concepts and topical issues in modern genetic epidemiology and highlights the issues facing researchers attempting to map and use genetic factors underlying common, complex human disease. The book is intended for advanced undergraduate and postgraduate students in public health, epidemiology, statistics, human genetics, clinical medicine or related disciplines. No specific specialist knowledge or technical background is assumed. In keeping with the broad readership that we anticipate for the book and the diverse background of people undertaking genetic epidemiological research, we provide introductory sections to equip readers with basic concepts and vocabulary. We anticipate that, depending on their professional background and specialist expertise, some readers may wish to skip some chapters.

In the first chapter, we provide an overall framework for investigating the role of familial factors, especially genetic determinants, in the causation of 'complex' human diseases such as diabetes and asthma. The chapter outlines the steps involved in integrating the biological science underlying modern genetics with the population science underpinning mainstream epidemiology. Chapter One also distinguishes the basic theory and methods of linkage studies and association studies. The second chapter provides an overview of linkage analysis and an introduction to family-based methods commonly used to map genetic loci that predispose to disease. Linkage analysis methods can be applied to both single gene disorders and complex diseases.

Chapter Three provides an overview of association analysis and discusses methods for the design and analysis of genetic association studies. Similarities between genetic association studies and classical epidemiological studies of environmental risk factors are discussed. Issues that are specific to studies of genetic risk factors such as the use of certain family-based designs are also discussed. Chapter Four extends this theme and reviews the state of knowledge about the structure of the human genome as related to single nucleotide polymorphisms (SNPs) and linkage disequilibrium, discusses the application of this knowledge to mapping complex disease genes using genome-wide association studies, and considers related methodological and study design issues. Chapter Five further discusses optimal study designs and the characteristics of a 'good' genetic association study. Across the world, such study design considerations have been partly responsible for a drive to invest substantial resources in the design and implementation of large-scale 'biobanks'. Biobanks are so called because they involve the systematic storage of biological material (for example blood or extracted DNA) and information from a large number of subjects, and may be disease-specific, exposure-orientated or population-based. Chapter Six discusses international biobanking initiatives and the rationale and issues around biobanking. Chapter Seven brings all the concepts discussed in the preceding chapters together to review the application of genetic epidemiology in population health, and discusses both the reality of genomic profiling and personalised medicine and the promise of new approaches, such as Mendelian randomisation.

Much of this book, in contrast to previous textbooks on genetic epidemiology, is focused on genetic association studies. Over the past decade, genetic epidemiology has experienced an important shift from family-based studies of genetic linkage to individual-based studies of genetic association. In part, this follows the recognition that for most common human diseases we are searching for common genetic variants of modest effect, and that such variants will be identified more easily using association studies. The shift to using association studies has been accompanied by an increasing methodological focus on optimal approaches to the design, analysis, meta-analysis and reporting of genetic association studies.

The past decade has been a tumultuous and exciting time in human genetics, and has seen the development of genetic epidemiology from an obscure body of knowledge to a key enabling discipline underpinning the mainstream of modern medical research. Explosive growth in technical capacity and genomic knowledge was tempered by initial failures to find genes for complex phenotypes using *any* strategy. Our statistical methods and ability to process data still lag far behind our ability to produce huge amounts of genomic data. What have we learned over the past decade of linkage mapping and association analyses? One important lesson is that everything in human genetics is context-specific – specific to the population, environmental exposures, genomic region and gene under investigation. There is no one paradigm for gene discovery and no single ideal study design or analytical approach. Despite a large number of reviews and ex cathedra statements on optimal study design and analytical strategies, it is clear that flexible, mixed approaches (often involving hypothesis-free designs) are desirable.

The genomics revolution has been accompanied by an unfortunate tendency to hyperbole. This has led to unrealistic expectations regarding the scope of deliverables and timeline for the integration of disease-gene discovery into clinical medicine, and to cynicism and pessimism within the genetics community. For genetic researchers, one of the most important tasks now is to not add to the hyperbole, but to establish and communicate realistic expectations. Nonetheless, the development of a consensus sequence of the entire human genome, the mapping of common SNPs, and cost-effective genotyping technologies leading to genome-wide association studies have combined convincingly in the past several years to demonstrate the feasibility of gene discovery for complex phenotypes and diseases. New genetic data combined with epidemiological data have delivered on their promise by enabling the identification of over 100 new, validated susceptibility genes for complex traits.

The major challenges facing most developed nations are those related to the high and, in some cases, rising prevalence of common, complex diseases, and the increasing complexity of their diagnosis, prevention and treatment. Such diseases are associated with substantial long-term morbidity and mortality and are major public health problems worldwide. Identification of causal genetic factors underlying common diseases is allowing fundamental insights into the biology of chronic disease, and this will in turn help to better define interventional, therapeutic and health promotion strategies (Khoury, 2004). The vital question for the coming decade is: how do we cost-effectively translate genomic findings into improved health outcomes? Even for situations such as type 2 diabetes, where spectacular advances have been made in the discovery of 11 common variants of modest effect explaining around 10% of disease risk (Lindgren and McCarthy, 2008), it is unclear how (or even whether) this information will be applied in direct clinical situations. This becomes even more acute in the realm of pharmacogenetic research, which has historically lagged behind complex gene discovery efforts. Reviews declaring that 'personalised medicine is almost here' or that 'individualised drug therapy will soon be a reality' should be treated with great caution (Nebert *et al.* 2008). It remains unclear whether personalised medicine or individualised drug therapy will ever be achievable by means of DNA testing alone. Yet it must be admitted that the current pace of change is so great in genomics and genetic epidemiology that it is hard to make firm predictions of any sort.

We hope that you find this book a useful and comprehensive introduction to the discipline of genetic epidemiology. For those of you go on to work in this field, we hope that you find it as exciting and fulfilling as we have.

References

Khoury MJ, (2004) The case for a global human genome epidemiology initiative. *Nat Genet*, 36, 1027-8.

Lindgren CM, McCarthy MI. (2008) Mechanisms of disease: genetic insights into the etiology of type 2 diabetes and obesity. *Nat Clin Pract Endocrinol Metab*, 4, 156-63.

Nebert DW, Zhang G, Vesell ES. (2008) From human genetics and genomics to pharmacogenetics and pharmacogenomics: past lessons, future directions. *Drug Metab Rev*, 40, 187-224.

ONE

Key concepts in genetic epidemiology

Paul R. Burton, Martin D. Tobin, John L. Hopper

Summary

This book provides an overview of central concepts and topical issues in modern genetic epidemiology. This chapter provides an overall framework for investigating the role of *familial* factors, especially genetic determinants, in the causation of complex human diseases such as diabetes. It outlines the steps involved in integrating the biological science underlying modern genetics with the population science underpinning mainstream epidemiology. In recognition of the diversity of readers' backgrounds, this chapter introduces basic concepts and vocabulary in genetic epidemiology. Some readers may wish to skip over some of this chapter, depending on their professional background and specialist expertise.

What is genetic epidemiology?

Epidemiology is usually defined as 'the study of the distribution, determinants [and control] of health–related states and events in populations'[1]. However, **genetic epidemiology** means different things to different people[2-7]. This book regards genetic epidemiology as[126]: 'A discipline closely allied to traditional epidemiology that focuses on the familial, and in particular genetic, determinants of disease and the joint effects of genes and non–genetic determinants. Crucially, *appropriate* account is taken of the biology that underlies the action of genes and the known mechanisms of inheritance'[8]. The word 'appropriate' is key – the manner in which the biology must be incorporated into any particular analysis varies markedly between studies and depends on the genetic information available.

Many genetic achievements to date have been based on monogenic, single–gene disorders[12] and have not required specialist input from genetic epidemiologists. However, investigations into the aetiological effect of genetic variants continue to evolve with advances in technology and biological knowledge. There is an increasing shift in focus from monogenic disorders to **complex disease**, which is characterised by a multitude of interacting genetic and environmental determinants[13;20]. Examples of complex diseases include diabetes mellitus, ischaemic heart disease, asthma and cancers[12;14-19].

Before information on DNA became available, scientists relating genetic variation to disease relied on the **presumed laws of inheritance**[8-11], which implied a biological model for the pattern of gene-sharing among close relatives. The next step was to assume a model for how a supposedly causative genetic variant might lead to disease – for example, the presence of two abnormal copies of 'gene G' may cause 'disease D'. This model could then be applied to an inheritance pattern and used to deduce causality from distribution of disease and trait aggregation within large families, or across groups of families. These types of investigations form the basis of **segregation analysis** and **genetic variance components analysis**, both of which are described later in this chapter.

As more information became known about the human *genome*, scientists focused on **genetic markers** – DNA sequences that vary from person to person[127]. Genetic markers can be localised to particular sites in the genome, but they are not necessarily responsible for determining health or disease. Scientists can estimate the likelihood of a causative genetic variant lying close to a particular genetic marker, and the distance to that marker, using a mathematical model. This model is based on the biology of **gamete formation** and **chromosomal recombination** and quantifies how often the marker is transmitted through a family in conjunction with an associated disease. The marker and the causative variant may or may not be within the same gene, and this forms the basis of **genetic linkage analysis** (see Chapter Two for more information). Genetic linkage analysis is the foundation of many breakthroughs in aetiological genetics, and is one of the most important and proven analytical tools available to the genetic epidemiologist when studying complex disease[127-131].

In the post-genomic era, extensive information about the human genome is available for use in genetic epidemiology studies. The first step is to deduce which of two versions of a potentially causative gene a given person possesses. The next step is to look for an association between variants in that gene and the disease of interest. In some respects, this analysis is fundamentally no different from a conventional epidemiological analysis of any disease-exposure association – often, there is no need to take particular account of the underlying biological model. However, a combined approach using both genetics and the inferential tools of modern epidemiology and biostatistics allows important aetiological questions to be addressed in ways that are more rigorous, and often more powerful, than approaches that fail to make optimal use of both disciplines. This concept will be an important and recurrent theme in this book.

In this chapter, the authors provide a framework for exploring the study design, analytical methods and challenges faced by the modern genetic epidemiologist. Figure 1.1 shows that a daunting investigation can be broken down into a series of manageable steps. It is not a prescriptive statement about how such research should be conducted – historical evidence, ease of recruiting study populations, and decreasing cost of genotyping are examples of 'modifying steps' in this study design pathway. Figure 1.1 does illustrate, however, that a proper understanding of the logical basis of each step helps to decide when short cuts are reasonable.

Figure 1.1: Schematic illustration of a systematic approach to the identification and characterisation of the genetic determinants of a complex disease

The cross on the lowest 'No' arrow indicates that it is probably illogical to stop trying to identify strong genetic determinants of disease simply because segregation analysis fails to provide significant evidence of a major gene.

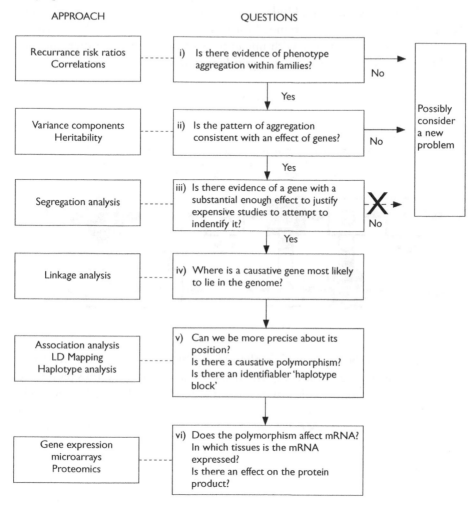

Genetics for genetic epidemiology

An understanding of basic genetics is essential for genetic epidemiologists. This section provides a brief overview of topics fundamental to genetic epidemiology. Words in the text that are highlighted in **_bold italics_** are defined in the Glossary at the end of this book. Readers familiar with contemporary human genetics may prefer to skip this section; those who are interested in a more comprehensive description of each concept are directed to relevant texts in the reference list[21;22].

DNA, RNA and proteins

The human genome is made up of **DNA** (deoxyribonucleic acid), which consists of a long sequence of *nucleotide* bases of four types: adenine (A), cytosine (C), guanine (G) and thymine (T). Under native conditions in the nucleus of a cell, DNA usually exists in double stranded form (Figure 1.2). Nucleotides of type A in one strand pair consistently with nucleotides of type T in the other, and the C and G nucleotides associate in an equivalent fashion, to form **base pairs** (bp).

Figure 1.2: Schematic diagram of double stranded DNA

Strong covalent bonds (indicated by diamonds) bind the DNA bases together along a single strand. Weaker hydrogen bonds result in the bases pairing up in a characteristic manner between the two strands. The base A consistently pairs with T, and the base C with G. The molecular structure of single stranded DNA allows two different ends called 5' and 3' (pronounced '5 prime' and '3 prime') to be identified, and the two strands are orientated in opposite directions.

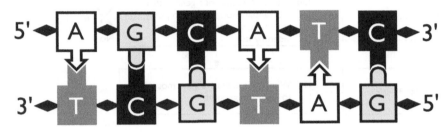

Double-stranded DNA is copied (**replicated**) by breaking apart the two single strands and constructing a new complementary strand for each one, thus producing two identical copies of the original double stranded DNA (Figure 1.3). A single strand of DNA can also act as a template to construct a complementary strand of a related molecule, called **RNA** (ribonucleic acid). This is known as **transcription**. RNA is similar to DNA, but has a slightly different molecular structure and the base of type T is replaced by one of type U (uracil; Figure 1.4).

In certain regions of the DNA known as **genes,** transcribed RNA encodes instructions that tell the cell how to assemble **amino acids** to make **proteins**.

Most genes contain alternating regions called **exons** and **introns**. Exons contain the protein coding sequences. The initial transcribed RNA molecule is complementary to the *whole* gene (both exons and introns). Post-transcriptional processing then produces mature **messenger RNA (mRNA)**, by excising and discarding the introns and splicing together the exons. This results in a single mRNA molecule that codes for a protein. The resultant production of protein molecules is called **translation**, and is followed by a series of post-translational processing steps.

Proteins fulfil a wide range of functions in the human body, such as the maintenance of structural integrity, catalysis of vital biochemical reactions, molecular transportation, biochemical signalling and various forms of bio-defence.

DNA sequence changes that influence health and disease generally exert an effect via changes in the functionality or availability of individual proteins.

Figure 1.3: Schematic illustration of DNA replication

The double stranded DNA (Figure 1.2) splits into two single strands. The two strands (top and bottom) are used as templates to re-synthesise new complementary second strands. The bases on the newly synthesised strands are indicated with stars. The full replication process results in duplicate copies of the original double stranded DNA.

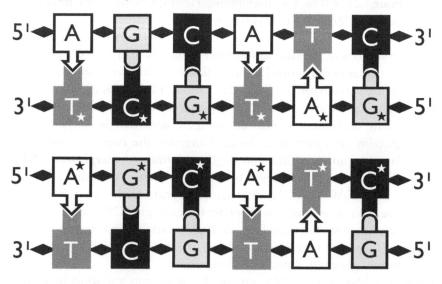

Figure 1.4: Schematic illustration of RNA transcription

The upper strand of the double stranded DNA is used as a template to synthesise a complementary RNA transcript. The RNA transcribed from the exonic regions of genes is then used as the basis of a translation template to assemble amino acids to form proteins.

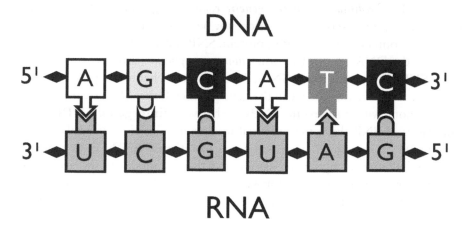

The human genome and variation in the DNA sequence

The complete DNA sequence in humans is referred to as the **human genome**, and the complete repertoire of proteins is known as the **human proteome**. The human genome is large – the *haploid* genome consists of approximately 3.3 billion bp. However, only around 3% of the genome consists of coding sequences[22] – the number of protein-coding genes was thought to be in the range 30,000-40,000[23-25] on completion of the first draft of the human genome, but this figure has now been revised to around 21,000 (www.ensembl.org/Homo_sapiens/index.html)[26; 132].

The vast majority (99.9%) of the genome is identical between any two unrelated individuals. However, there are many ways in which the DNA sequence can vary between two versions of the same chromosome. The alternative DNA sequences found at a particular chromosomal location (*locus*) are known as *alleles*.

DNA sequence variants can be classified in various ways[22]. Classification criteria include: the physical nature of the DNA sequence variation; the impact that the variant may have on protein formation; and more generally, the variant's effect upon susceptibility to a particular disease. Currently, the two most important structural classes are *microsatellites* and *single nucleotide polymorphisms* (*SNPs*).

Microsatellites are multiple repeats of a short sequence, typically 2-8 bp in length, such as 'CACACACA…' (a dinucleotide repeat). Alleles are differentiated by the number of repeats they incorporate; for example, 'CA_{12}' would denote 12 CA repeats in a row. Microsatellites are highly variable and most people are *heterozygous* (they have two different alleles) at any given locus. Microsatellite sequences are not generally found in coding regions.

In contrast, a SNP is as a DNA variant that represents variation in a single nucleotide. As of April 2009, there were almost 18 million known SNPs with a unique position in the human genome, with over 6.5 million independently validated (dbSNP build 130 at www.ncbi.nlm.nih.gov/projects/SNP/snp_summary.cgi). The large number of validated SNPs, in addition to their ease of typing, has resulted in the widespread use of SNPs analysis in genetic epidemiology, despite the fact that individual SNPs may carry limited information.[25]

As a result of *redundancy in the genetic code*, changes in the DNA coding sequence in a protein-coding region do not necessarily lead to changes in the amino acid content of the resulting protein. SNPs occurring in protein–coding regions of the DNA are termed either *non-synonymous* (also known as coding SNPs, *cSNPs*[25]) or *synonymous* SNPs, depending on whether they do or do not modify the amino acid sequence in the gene product. Other SNPs lie in the non-coding regions within (**intronic SNPs**) or between (**intergenic SNPs**) genes.

All classes of SNPs have the potential to alter the function or availability of a protein. When they do, they are known as **functional SNPs**. For example, a SNP could alter transcription regulation and thereby modulate the availability of a critical protein. However, a non-synonymous SNP in a coding sequence is more likely to be functional than most other classes of SNP[25]. Many of the genetic variants that have been discovered to underlie **Mendelian** (single gene) disorders are functional SNPs. In the realm of complex human disease, although dramatic progress has been made in defining reproducible statistical associations arising from genome-wide association scans, the true distribution of disease-associated variants between non-coding and coding sequences remains speculative[25; 133-135] (see Chapters Three and Four).

Chromosomes, gamete formation and recombination

The human genome is distributed among 46 **chromosomes** comprising 23 **homologous chromosome pairs**. There are 22 pairs of autosomes, numbered 1–22, and one pair of **sex chromosomes** ('X,X' in a female and 'X,Y' in a male). The complete set of chromosomes is termed the **diploid** complement, designated '46,XX' in females and '46,XY' in males. For any individual, one chromosome in each homologous pair is derived from the mother and one comes from the father. With the exception of the 'X' and 'Y' chromosomes in a male, two homologous homologous chromosomes each have the same basic structure, including the same gene sequence in the same positions along their length. However, two homologous chromosomes can generally be distinguished from each other by sequence variations at numerous loci.

Meiosis is the process of cell division and accompanying replication and partitioning of DNA, leading to the formation of **gametes** (sperm and ova). This process commences with the full diploid chromosome complement. As each gamete is formed it receives, at random, one member of each homologous chromosomal pair. This means that gametes each have a haploid genome: ova are '23,X' and sperm are either '23,X' or '23,Y'. Sperm and ova fuse to produce a **zygote**, which matures into a human embryo and has a diploid genome. A complete description of meiosis can be found in Strachan & Read[22].

One might deduce that there is a 50% probability that any given gamete receives one particular chromosome from a homologous pair, and that there are a total of 2^{23} distinct gametes that can be produced by an individual. However, during gamete formation, homologous chromosomes align but do not get directly transmitted to the gamete as whole chromosomes. **Crossover** events result in a chromosome that is transmitted to a gamete as a *mixture* of the two homologous chromosomes (Figure 1.5). Crossovers can split up alleles that that lie together along a common parental chromosome (at different loci) and can also cause alleles that originally came from different grandparents to appear on the same chromosome. These processes are jointly known as **recombination**.

Traditional gene mapping methods make use of recombination. If two genes are very close together on one chromosome, the chance of a crossover occurring between them is very small. An odd number of crossovers results in recombination – as the distance between genes increases, the probability of an odd number of crossovers between them rises to a maximum of 50%. An estimate of the proportion of meioses actually resulting in a recombination (recombination fraction), can be used to approximate the distance between two genes on the human genome.

Figure 1.5: Crossing over and recombination

Two hypothetical loci, U and V, are sited 20% and 30% along the length of chromosome 14. They existed as alleles U_1 and V_7 on chromosome 14_{PAT} (the chromosome derived originally from the father's father) and alleles U_3 and V_4 on chromosome 14_{MAT} (the chromosome derived originally from the father's mother). Given crossovers at 23% and 59% along chromosome 14, one obtains the two 'mixed chromosome 14s' of the father illustrated in the centre. In this case, it is the right-hand chromosome that is transmitted to the gamete, and this has alleles U_3 and V_7. These two alleles were independently derived from the father's mother and the father's father, respectively.

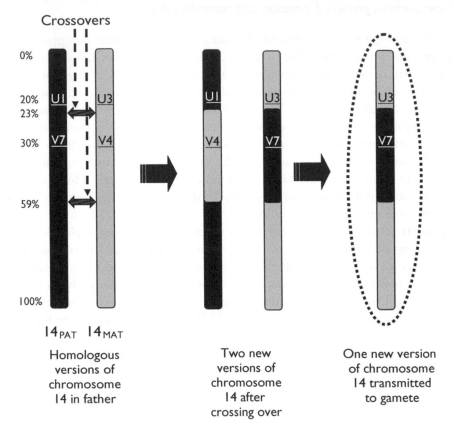

Distance along a chromosome is measured in **centimorgans (cM)**, where 1 cM corresponds, on average, to approximately one million bp[27]. The exact relationship between cM and bp varies between males and females and also depends on the location within the genome. An estimate of recombination fraction can also be mathematically transformed into an expected number of crossover events.

Genotypes, haplotypes and phenotypes

Although the term **genotype** is sometimes used to refer to the *overall* genetic constitution of an individual[22], this usage is rare in genetic epidemiology. In this book, genotype refers to the genetic constitution of an individual at a particular locus. For example, imagine there are three loci U,V and W lying on a chromosome, and the alleles U_3–V_2–W_2 lie along one homologous chromosome and U_1–V_2–W_1 along the other. The genotypes of the individual at the U,V and W loci would then be U_1U_3, V_2V_2 and W_1W_2, respectively. Expressed in this manner, a genotype has no natural order and $U_1U_3 = U_3U_1$. Consequently, if the two homologous chromosomes had carried alleles U_1–V_2–W_2 and U_3–V_2–W_1, then the genotypes would still be U_1U_3, V_2V_2 and W_1W_2.

The allelic configuration along a single chromosome is called a ***haplotype*** and, unlike genotypes, haplotypes obviously *are* dependent on the actual order of alleles on the chromosome. The haplotype information in a parent also implies the ***phase*** of that parent's meioses[27], as it indicates the presence or absence of recombination.

This book uses the term ***phenotype*** interchangeably with ***trait*** to refer to measurable characteristics of an individual, other than genotypes[22]. Phenotypes may be **binary disease states** – the presence or absence of asthma, for example, or **quantitative characteristics** such as systolic blood pressure. Some simple binary phenotypes are only **expressed** (present) if there are two copies of an abnormal allele at a causative locus (an example of this is found in cystic fibrosis). The abnormal allele is described as ***recessive*** in causing this particular phenotype. Other abnormal phenotypes may be expressed fully in the presence of a single copy of the abnormal allele, even if the allele on the homologous chromosome is entirely normal. In this instance, the abnormal allele is dominant for the trait.

These two deterministic situations are extremes and, in reality, there is often an intermediate state. The probability of a given phenotype being expressed in a subject with a particular genotype is termed ***penetrance***. ***Co-dominance*** refers to a heterozygote penetrance that is intermediate between that of the corresponding homozygotes – that is, neither phenotype is dominant, and both are expressed in this individual (for example, as found in the molecular expression of sickle cell trait). Penetrance can also be modelled in terms of age-at-onset distribution by genotype, if the expression of a trait is age-dependent. These concepts apply to a trait defined either by an ungrouped quantitative scale or by coarsely grouped categories in an ordinal scale.

The fusion of genetics and epidemiology

Phenotypic aggregation within families

It is important to distinguish between the clinical term **familial clustering**, which indicates extended families that happen to have multiple cases of a particular disease or syndrome, and the epidemiological term **familial aggregation**. Familial aggregation refers to a greater frequency, on average, of a disease among close relatives of individuals *with* the disease than among relatives of individuals *without* the disease.

In mainstream epidemiology, the family unit is given the same consideration as other clustering units during simple analyses of familial aggregation. In identifying phenotypic aggregation within families, there is no attempt made to determine the mechanistic origin of this aggregation[136].

Binary traits

Familial aggregation is often assessed for binary traits (such as diabetes mellitus) using the **recurrence risk ratio**[30] (a ratio of *prevalences*, λ_R) or an allied measure[31]. Prevalence refers to 'the proportion of a population that has a [particular] disease at a specific point in time'[32] and is a measure of the existence of disease at the time of baseline assessment, rather than of newly occurring disease arising after that assessment.

The pattern of recurrence risk ratios across different types of relatives can provide valuable information regarding the origin of a binary trait[30] and can be used to augment the statistical power of *linkage* studies[14].

The equation:

<Eqn>

$$\hat{\lambda}_R = \frac{\hat{P}_R}{\hat{P}}$$

represents the estimated recurrence risk ratio in relatives of type R, where $\hat{P}_R$ is the estimated prevalence of disease in relatives of class R of affected cases, and $\hat{P}$ is the estimated prevalence in the general population. λ_S is used to denote the estimated prevalence of disease among siblings of affected cases[14].

Estimating prevalence can be difficult and entails consideration of several non-trivial issues. First, assessment of the disease (phenotype) must be done very carefully, and must include disease definition, age at onset and duration of disease[33]. Second, the study sample should be properly representative of the target population, and subjects with disease must not be systematically over- or under-recruited. Avoiding bias may require investment of substantial resources to ensure a sufficiently high response rate.

In genetic epidemiology, as in mainstream epidemiology, it is often difficult to obtain a representative or random sample of the general population that is large enough to guarantee adequate statistical power. Consequently, families are often recruited *because* they have affected members. This is known as **outcome-based sampling**, which is often more informative, increases power, and has obvious benefits for estimating λ_R.

However, outcome-based sampling may lead to severe ascertainment bias[34] because the trait's familial determinants are typically unobserved in a study of familial aggregation and that those 'at risk' families that, by chance, have no affected members will be missed from any analysis. Furthermore, the data used to estimate P_R can take diverse form[34]. The consequences of any non-random sampling method must be considered carefully, and bias accounted for during analysis[34-44]. Expert advice should be sought where necessary.

Equal deliberation should apply to other measures of familial aggregation, and to **variance components models** and **segregation models** used to investigate patterns of aggregation within families[36-39;43;44]. These models are discussed later in this chapter.

There are three important interpretational issues that warrant emphasis. First, the incidence (and hence prevalence) of many complex diseases increases steeply with age, whereas λ_R often declines[45]. The age distribution of both the general population and of the subjects' relatives must be scrutinised and, at the very least, adjustments made for any differences between the two. Second, if a phenotype is common, λ_R can only take a small value, even if every available relative is affected. An example of common phenotypes with $\hat{P} = 0.5$ (implying that $\hat{\lambda}_R$ cannot be greater than 2) are some measures of skin prick sensitivity to common allergens[46]. Hence caution is required when comparing λ_R across different diseases or contexts. Third, λ_R measures the combined impact of *all* causes of familial aggregation, and not just that of genes[14; 30].

There are a number of different approaches that approximate the relative risk of disease for the relatives of an affected individual, when compared to the risk for the general population. These approaches are generally referred to as **familial relative risk**. In addition to the λ_R-based methods just described, there are others based on incidence rate ratios derived from longitudinal *cohort studies* (with or without standardisation)[47]. Risch reviews these techniques[45].

Quantitative traits

Intra-family correlation co-efficient (ICC) and other correlation or covariance-based measures are commonly used to assess familial aggregation of a continuous trait, such as (untreated) blood pressure. This approach to genetic analysis dates back more than a century to Francis Galton[48;49] and Karl Pearson[50]. ICC is the proportion of a phenotype's *total* variability that is reasonably attributable to *real* variability between families[51]. The larger the ICC, the greater the intra-familial aggregation. In essence, a genetic epidemiological assessment of aggregation for a continuous measure is fundamentally no different from, and may be viewed as predating[10;49], analogous problems in traditional epidemiology and social science[51;52].

Consequently, all relevant techniques from these disciplines can be used in genetic epidemiology, including linear regression, analysis of variance, generalised estimating equations, multi-level modelling, structural equation modelling and generalised linear mixed modelling,[51-57]. As with the assessment of a binary phenotype aggregation, non-random ascertainment can seriously bias an ICC[42].

Interpretation

For many complex diseases, including cancers, heart disease, asthma and osteoporosis, the average familial relative risk in first-degree relatives is around 2.0[45]. Risk tends to be greater in affected individuals with a young age at onset[45], falls as the familial relationship becomes more distant[30], and increases with a higher number of affected relatives. Although a familial relative risk of 2.0 may seem to be modest in conventional epidemiological terms, it does imply that there could be both genetic or non-genetic familial risk factors of at least an order of magnitude stronger[58;59].

This effect strengthens with the rarity of the causative factor. For example, dominant alleles of the *BRCA1* gene affect approximately 1 in 500 women, and result in a 10- to 20-fold increase in the risk of breast cancer. However, this produces only a small increased risk of disease in first-degree relatives across the population (λ_R is about 1.1). A λ_R of around 2.0 might also indicate several common alleles that are each associated with a slightly lower relative risk. Knowing only the λ_R does not reveal the most likely genetic or familial model.

A simple assessment of familial aggregation is not focused on biological factors, so evidence of familial aggregation does not necessarily imply genetic effects. Nevertheless, for many complex diseases, the known non-genetic risk factors appear to have a minor effect and do not appear to explain familial aggregation adequately. For example, parity (number of children born), age at menarche, age at menopause and body mass index increase the risk of breast cancer in first-degree relatives by less than 5%[59]. But these factors may well be surrogates for stronger, more fundamental determinants not yet identifiable by current methods. Environmental and lifestyle risk factors are often measured by questionnaire and may be subject to substantial measurement errors, which can lead to an underestimate of effect size and of familial correlation. Therefore, the non-genetic contribution to risk, and to estimated correlation between relatives, may be markedly understated.

Explanation for the pattern of aggregation

Variance components modelling

To estimate genetic contribution to identified familial aggregation, the epidemiological analysis must include a biological model with two important elements. The first is a logical representation of precisely how a phenotype might be modulated by one or more genes, such as the **additive genetic effect model** (Box 1.1)[10;60;61]. The second element is a mathematical model quantifying the probabilities of sharing alleles **identical by descent (IBD)** (Box 1.2) among different classes of relatives. Incorporation of both of these elements into an appropriate mathematical model, such as a **hierarchical variance components**

model[54;56;60;61], enables measurement of genetic variability consistent with the observed familial variability patterns in the phenotype.

It is important to note that an apparently robust model does not exclude the existence of another genetic or non-genetic model that fits equally well. This approach can be extended to include the covariance or correlation patterns, or both, that would be expected for other, more complex models of genetic determination – for example, including **genetic dominance** (see Chapter Three) in addition to additive genetic effects[10;54;60-63]. Analysis can also include the correlation or covariance patterns caused by unmeasured environmental determinants shared by a whole family, or just by siblings, as well as determinants that vary as individuals live together and apart[29;54;56;60;61;63]. Finally, many environmental and lifestyle *exposures* are unique to an individual. These factors do *not* contribute to the covariance between relatives, but they do affect the total variability of a quantitative trait, thereby reducing correlations. Significant methodological developments in this area have come from the analysis of twin studies[9;54;64;65;66].

One important point that is often misunderstood is that variance components analyses of the type described here do *not* require information about characterised genotypes or measured environmental determinants. In other words, they facilitate indirect investigation of genetic effects without the need for taking blood and analysing DNA. However, if information regarding specific genes and environmental determinants is available, then this should be added to an appropriate variance components model. Box 1.3 discusses variance components models that are most commonly used in genetic epidemiology.

Box 1.1: Additive genetic effects

One of the simplest paradigms for the effect of genes on a continuous complex trait is the **additive genetic effects model**[10;29;60;6;63]. Under this model, there are assumed to be an unspecified number (one, several or many) of genes that influence the trait. Each of these is assumed to have an unspecified number of alleles. The model of additive effects simply implies that a given allele at a given locus adds a constant to, or subtracts a constant from, the expected value of the trait. The amount added or subtracted varies in an unknown way between alleles and between loci. For example, one of a number of relevant genes may be called G and it may have four different alleles: G_1 adds three to the trait; G_2 adds six; G_3 subtracts two; and G_4 adds one. Under the model of additive genetic effects, the contribution of the G gene to the expected value of the trait in an individual who is of genotype G_1G_2 is +9, while for a subject of genotype G_3G_4 it is −1. Critically, under this model, the effect that any one allele exerts is assumed to be the same *regardless* of which allele it is paired with. Thus G_1 adds three regardless of whether the genotype is G_1G_1 (**+3 +3** = +6), G_1G_2 (**+3 +6** = +9), G_1G_3 (**+3** −2 = +1), or G_1G_4 (**+3** +1 = +4). One of the reasons that this model is so widely used is that unless there is a *marked* departure from this assumption – for example, if G_1 adds six if paired with G_2 but subtracts three if paired with G_3 (an example of genetic dominance as described in Chapter Three) – then the additive model will usually capture much of the aetiological information that can be reasonably explained by genes. In addition, the model is mathematically straightforward. Fisher[10] shows that the model implies that genes make a contribution to the variability of the trait, such that the genetically mediated covariance between two subjects is directly proportional to the proportion of alleles they share **identical by descent** (Box 1.2 and Table 1.1). Covariance[57] is a statistical measure of the tendency to similarity between two individuals.

Table 1.1: Characteristic IBD sharing for different categories of relative pair on the assumption that parents are unrelated

	Parents	Parent and child	Full siblings	Grandparent and grandchild	Uncle and niece	First cousins	Half siblings	Identical twins
Probability of 2 alleles shared IBD	0	0	0.25	0	0	0	0	1
Probability of 1 allele shared IBD	0	1	0.5	0.5	0.5	0.25	0.5	0
Probability of 0 alleles shared IBD	1	0	0.25	0.5	0.5	0.75	0.5	0
Proportion of alleles shared IBD	Exactly 0	Exactly 0.5	On average 0.5	On average 0.25	On average 0.25	On average 0.125	On average 0.25	Exactly 1

The upper three rows denote the expected probability with which two relatives of the designated category share two, one or zero alleles at any given autosomal locus.

Box 1.2: Identity by descent (IBD) and identity by state (IBS)

If two parents are both of genotype G_1G_2 at a given locus on an autosome, then two of their offspring – full siblings each of genotype G_1G_2 – may have received their G_1 alleles from the same parent, for example both from the mother, or one from either parent. Further, if the G_1 alleles are from different parents then so are the G_2 alleles. This means that the two siblings may have either inherited the *same* two alleles from both parents (Case A: both received the mother's G_1 and the father's G_2 or both received the mother's G_2 and the father's G_1) or they may have inherited *different* alleles from the two parents (Case B: one sibling received the mother's G_1 and the father's G_2 while the other received the mother's G_2 and the father's G_1). These statements introduce the key concepts of identity by descent (IBD) and identity by state (IBS).

Any two individuals with genotypes G_1G_2 are said to share two alleles IBS. This is true regardless of the origin of the two alleles, and regardless of whether or not the two individuals are relatives. Similarly, any two subjects with genotypes G_1G_2 and G_2G_5 are said to share one allele IBS. Thus, the two siblings in the preceding paragraph share two alleles IBS in both Case A and Case B.

In contrast, an allele can only be said to be shared IBD by two individuals if it has been inherited *directly* from a common ancestor, which may be one of the two individuals themselves. Importantly, it is excess IBD sharing that differentiates relatives from unrelated individuals, and it is IBD sharing that is generally of primacy in genetic epidemiology. Table 1.1 illustrates the characteristic IBD sharing for a variety of classes of relative. The two siblings in the first paragraph of this Box share two alleles IBD in Case A and no alleles IBD in Case B.

Theoretically, many structurally identical alleles can be traced back to a common ancestor many generations ago and so, in part, IBS reflects a mixture of IBD over several generations. However, even given a common ancestor only five generations back, the probability of two apparently unrelated individuals in the present generation sharing any one allele IBD at a given locus is less than 1 in 500. Except in genetically isolated populations, systematic IBD sharing between apparently unrelated individuals will also have little impact on the correlation or covariance structure.

Although the difference between IBS and IBD is central to understanding techniques such as linkage analysis and variance components analysis, it is less important in association analysis, particularly in those situations where all relevant genotypes are observed directly and the ancestral origin of each allele is irrelevant (see Box 1.4).

> **Box 1.3:** Common approaches to the fitting of variance components models
>
> **Variance components analysis** can be undertaken using conventional statistical models, which use optimisation procedures such as maximum likelihood[62] and generalised least squares[54], or Markov chain Monte Carlo based approaches such as Gibbs sampling[56]. Among genetic epidemiologists, an example of traditional approaches to aid the specification of these models is **path analysis**, invented by Sewall Wright nearly 100 years ago[120]. These models are often fitted using structural equation modelling in LISREL or Mx[54;121]. Variance components models can also be fitted using sophisticated maximum likelihood engines such as FISHER[122]. The underlying models are fundamentally similar, regardless how they may be specified[60], and it is entirely appropriate to fit these same models in statistical environments more familiar to non-genetic epidemiologists. These include: multilevel modelling in MLWin[123]; generalised estimating equations in any one of a number of standard packages that support them[53]; and generalised linear mixed modelling in WinBUGS[56;124]. The use of these flexible modelling environments means that if there *is* information available on characterised genotypes, measured environmental determinants or known demographics, these can be included in the analysis as conventional regression covariates. Equivalent approaches can also be used for binary phenotypes[54;56;69] and for traits that can best be expressed as a survival time[94;125], such as an age at onset or age at death.

Heritability

One of the principal reasons for fitting a variance components model is to estimate the variance attributable to *additive* **genetic effects (S^2_A)**. This reflects the component of the **total phenotypic variance (S^2_T)** that is attributed to unmeasured additive genetic effects (Box 1.1), after adjusting for measured genetic and non-genetic determinants. **Narrow sense heritability** is equal to S^2_A/S^2_T – that is, the proportion of total phenotypic variance due to additive genetic effects[137]. Certain family studies, especially those of monozygous (identical) twins, also allow estimation of the **phenotypic variance attributable to *all* genetic effects (S^2_G),** including non-additive effects at individual loci (**dominance variance**) and between loci (**epistatic variance**) (see Chapter Three for more information). **Broad sense heritability (H^2_B)** is defined as S^2_G/S^2_T [137].

Heritability is a beguiling concept open to misinterpretation. It is not about causation per se, but rather the causes of variation in a trait of interest, in a defined population, at a particular point in time[10;29;67]. Fisher[68] points out that whereas S^2_A has a simple genetic meaning, the S^2_T is a complex 'hotch-potch' construct that fuses genetic variance, the variance resulting from a shared environment, and residual variance due to both unshared and unmeasured determinants and to measurement error. Thus the heritability for any given phenotype may vary quite markedly between, and even within, different settings[7;67].

Heritability is formally defined for quantitative traits[67]. For binary traits, it may be derived via a hypothetical construct called **liability** applied in a version of variance components modelling. Liability is an underlying, unobservable, normally distributed quantitative trait that is assumed to determine the probability of an individual developing the disease of interest[69;70;61;67]. Unfortunately, the key assumption – that liability is normally distributed in a binary disease state – is untestable[67]. Furthermore, the heritability of liability is neither clearly defined nor interpreted[29;71;45;72;73]. The principal reason for calculating heritability for a quantitative trait, rather than quoting a raw value for variance due to additive genetic effects, is that heritability standardises S^2_A for the intrinsic variability of the phenotypic trait. This is of obvious scientific utility. However, the intrinsic variability of a binary phenotype is determined chiefly by the **binomial error**, which is fixed mathematically. For most complex traits, the intrinsic variability will also include random, unshared errors that contribute directly to the assumed liability and are specific to an individual. For studies involving a single measurement of the binary trait, the additional variability arising from these error terms is generally not identifiable[56]. Consequently, the variance of liability is fixed by assumption and not from the data. There would seem to be little value in standardising S^2_A for an assumed quantity, which suggests that calculating the heritability of a binary trait is somewhat redundant in this situation.

The media, and some scientists, sometimes refer to heritability as 'the extent to which a trait is caused by genetic factors'. This view is incorrect. If a trait is dependent on the presence of an allele for which the entire population is homozygous, variation at that locus will not affect the observed variance of the trait, the liability of disease or heritability. For example, the fact that most humans have two arms is clearly determined primarily by the human genome, but genetic variation accounts for very little of the variance of number of arms within the general population. Similarly, a near ubiquitous environmental exposure will have little or no effect on S^2_T. Selection of covariates into an adjustment model also influences interpretation – for example, adjustment for an important environmental covariate might well decrease S^2_T but leave S^2_A unchanged, thus apparently increasing narrow sense heritability. For these reasons, it is often preferable to quote the magnitude of the variance components (such as S^2_A) individually, rather than relying solely on the overall heritability value[68]. The individual variance components each have a direct scientific interpretation, and their estimates can be compared meaningfully within and between populations[56;74].

Readers may wonder why genetic epidemiologists bother to calculate heritability, if it has so many pitfalls. One reason is that most studies' power for discovering genes is positively associated with the heritability of the trait of interest – selecting a study population with a high heritability may enhance analytical efficiency. Moreover, knowledge of a trait's high heritability supports proposals for a study investigating the genetic determinants of that trait. Conversely, low heritability may indicate to the study's investigators and funding bodies that genetic effects may be difficult to find. In either case, interpretation demands expert understanding of the nature of the trait.

Justification for expensive studies

Is there any evidence of genes with a large enough effect to justify the expensive studies that try to find them? This question is addressed by **segregation analysis**[29;75;76], which assesses genetic variants – regardless of how rare – that have a strong effect on disease susceptibility, and whose Mendelian segregation within families explains a substantial part of that trait's familial aggregation. This information is useful in its own right[77], or it may be used to generate estimates for a **parametric linkage analysis**[78] (see Chapter Two for more information).

Segregation analysis is defined by Elston[79] as 'the statistical methodology used to determine from family data the mode of inheritance of a particular phenotype, especially with a view to elucidating [major] gene effects'. The author emphasises that segregation analysis considers four things: (1) the genotypic distribution of mating individuals; (2) the relationship between phenotype and genotype; (3) the mode of inheritance; and (4) the sampling scheme[79]. Although computationally demanding, it is now possible to fit models that estimate allele frequencies and risk functions, and that include more than one mode of inheritance. This is provisional on the available family structures being adequately informative (as Cui *et al.* note[80]).

As with variance components analysis, classical segregation analysis has no requirement for observed genotypes. It may be viewed as a special investigation of familial aggregation, sometimes focusing on the pattern of aggregation *within individual families*, rather than averaging patterns across the population. It is worth noting that the results of a segregation analysis can be very sensitive to inappropriate ascertainment adjustment[38].

Several factors affect the extent to which a major gene is worthy of biological investigation. These include: the prevalence of the deleterious variant(s); the epidemiological characteristics of any resulting disease; and the strengths of additional genetic and environmental determinants. The potential clinical or public health value must also be considered. These are important issues and will be discussed further in Chapter Seven on Mendelian randomisation. The ability of segregation analysis to detect a major gene effect is also a function of the quantity, quality and structure of the family data that are available. In light of these uncertainties, it might be viewed as irrational *not* to progress further investigation of a putative gene effect simply because a segregation analysis has failed to provide evidence for a major gene (Figure 1.1).

Segregation analyses have been used less often since the start of the modern genomic revolution and the focus on complex human disease. This decline is partly due to concurrent increases in computational power that enable **parametric linkage models** (see Chapter Two) to assume a wide variety of different inheritance models, and a range of values for additional genetic parameters. Another reason is that contemporary genetic linkage analyses are often based on **non-parametric methods**, and therefore do not require parameter estimates for a specific genetic model obtained from segregation analyses. The overriding reason, however, is that segregation analyses that assume one major genetic factor seldom make sense in the context of complex human diseases that involve multiple, interacting genetic and environmental factors of generally modest effect on phenotype[138].

Location of a causative gene

Having obtained evidence of a likely genetic contribution to complex disease – without genotyping – the next step is to locate and identify any causative genes. One option is to proceed immediately to studying the direct effects of the genes identified (this is discussed in the section on association analysis later in this chapter). However, most complex diseases have multiple *candidate genes*, the normal and abnormal effects of which are often unknown. Therefore, candidate gene work is often preceded or paralleled by an attempt to localise relevant regions of the genome.

Genetic linkage analysis has been used successfully to locate major genes for many monogenic conditions[12]. However, there have been far fewer successes analysing complex disease[81;82], mainly owing to severe limitations in statistical power (see Chapter Two for a detailed discussion of this issue). Most true effect sizes tend to be small when averaged across the population; complex phenotypes are often multidimensional and subject to substantial measurement error; there is marked aetiological heterogeneity; and the measurable predictive variables may not be strongly associated with the actual causative agent(s)[139].

Genetic linkage analysis is possibly the best example of a common investigative approach in genetic epidemiology derived almost entirely from consideration of the underlying genetics. There are no corresponding tools in traditional behavioural and environmental epidemiology, although there are clear parallels in other specialised epidemiological fields such as infectious disease epidemiology. Genetic linkage analysis relies entirely on the tendency for short regions of the genome to be passed on to the next generation intact[78;83-85] – that is, without being subject to a recombination event at meiosis. A marker that is passed down through a family and is consistently associated with the disease of interest suggests that there is a gene with a functional effect located close to that marker.

Focus placed on the genetics of complex disease should not obscure the importance of clinical knowledge accrued over many years. The identification of familial syndromes has been critical to the success of linkage studies, because often an attempt has been made to reduce the complex disease to one of its monogenic forms. One example is the syndrome of bowel cancer, which led to the identification of the role of *mutations* in DNA mismatch repair genes in disposing individuals to cancer[86-88]. This was historically referred to as hereditary non-polyposis colorectal cancer or Lynch syndrome[89]. Other notable examples include the familial breast-ovary syndrome that led to the cloning of *BRCA1*[90], and the female and male breast cancer syndrome that led to the cloning of *BRCA2*[91].

Association analysis

Traditional epidemiology often attempts to ascertain across a study population, whether a measured environmental exposure is consistently associated with an observed disease. **Association analysis** in genetic epidemiology seeks to identify disease association with measured genetic exposures – the alleles of genotyped genes[140]. This approach is akin to traditional epidemiology being applied to genotypes or alleles across a population (Box 1.4). Many of the analytical approaches used in epidemiology and medical statistics – univariate methods and regression analysis[57;92;93], for example – can be applied directly to association analyses in genetic epidemiology. Furthermore, the models discussed in Box 1.3 can be easily extended to accommodate data that has complex correlation structure, including family data; longitudinal data; data naturally subject to geographical or temporal clustering; and/or data collected under a multi-stage sampling scheme. All these

---

Box 1.4: A simple association analysis

The simplest class of association analysis involves a binary disease trait and a putative functional gene with two alleles (G_1 and G_2). This requires a study dataset consisting of an adequate number of unrelated individuals, each of whom has been genotyped for the gene of interest and can be classified as having, or not having, the disease of interest. The easiest approach is then to construct a conventional **2×3 contingency table**, with rows representing disease status and columns representing the three possible genotypes: G_1G_1, G_1G_2 and G_2G_2.

	G_1G_1	G_1G_2	G_2G_2
Disease	109	118	26
No disease	138	88	21

This table can be analysed in whatever manner is desired. In this example, the analytical focus is on the **distribution of genotypes by disease status** (see Chapter Three for details of analyses based on the allele distribution). A conventional χ^2 test for association takes the value $\chi^2_{[2\ df]} = 8.23$ ($p = 0.016$), implying 'significant' heterogeneity in the risk of disease associated with the three genotypes. A χ^2 test for linear trend is obtained as $\chi^2_{[1\ df]} = 6.23$ ($p = 0.013$). Alternatively, if the table is analysed using **logistic regression**, it can be estimated that, on average, each additional copy of the G_2 allele increases the odds of disease by a multiplicative factor of 1.41 (95% confidence interval 1.07 to 1.85).

How the results of such analyses should be interpreted is critically dependent on whether one is conducting a one-off test on a single candidate gene, when the analysis can be interpreted at face value, or whether this is merely one marker gene among many that are being tested as part of a whole-genome scan. The latter situation calls for a demanding adjustment and the extremely low a priori probability that a given locus is truly associated with the disease[15;16;18]. Chapter Three outlines these issues in further detail.

---

concepts can also be generalised to a variety of phenotypic classes, including binary traits; continuous normally distributed traits; and time-to-event (survival time) analyses[53;54;94].

Association analysis will be discussed further in Chapters Three, Four and Five, but it is important to note that although association analysis is essentially traditional epidemiology applied to genetic exposure variables, there are several biological features that are crucial to a full understanding of allelic association. First and most fundamental is that a test of association may be informative even when based on non-functional genetic variants. This is because the association could be **indirect** –that is, due to **linkage disequilibrium (LD)** (Box 1.5) between a disease susceptibility *polymorphism* and a non-functional marker gene (see Chapter Three)[19;95;96]. Indirect association analysis based on LD allows finer mapping than conventional linkage analysis: LD allows one to infer the position of the disease to within about 1cM (1 million base pairs) either side of the marker[27], whereas it may be difficult for conventional linkage analysis to locate a complex trait within 10 cM[141].

Box 1.5: Linkage disequilibrium in contrast to simple linkage

Imagine a functional gene D, affecting a binary disease trait of interest that lies 0.01 cM (about 10 kilobases) away from a known marker. Let us assume that, 2,000 generations ago, a new deleterious mutation D* appeared in a single individual on a chromosome that happened to carry the allele M_{17} at that marker. Any individual carrying D* now will have inherited the relevant part of the original disease-bearing chromosome via an inheritance pathway involving 2,000 meioses. Given the stated physical distance between the marker and the disease gene, the probability of a crossover occurring between the two at any one meiosis will be 0.0001 and the probability that *no* crossover will have occurred in any of the 2,000 meioses will be $(1-0.0001)^{2000} \approx 0.82$. This may well make it possible to detect a population-wide association between the disease and the M_{17} allele of the marker, even though M_{17} has nothing to do with the aetiology of the disease. This is known as **linkage disequilibrium (LD)**. See Chapter Three for a more detailed consideration of the theory underpinning the analysis and interpretation of LD.

LD implies linkage between two loci that is so tight that it leads to an association at a population level. This is in contrast to simple linkage, where the two loci tend to be further apart and there is a greater chance of recombination occurring at any single meiosis. In simple linkage, a disease-causing variant may be closely associated with a particular marker allele, say M_3, in one family, but may be equally closely associated with M_8 in a second family and M_1 in a third family. The 'within-family associations' over a small number of generations are strong and consistent, but there is no systematic association across the population as a whole. LD is important because it allows much finer mapping than simple linkage, and is therefore a sensible intermediate between coarse mapping using simple linkage and expensive molecular work that characterises individual candidate genes in a much smaller region.

The International HapMap Project (www.hapmap.org) was a major collaborative initiative to map out regions of LD and to 'develop a haplotype map of the human genome' [97] (see also Chapter Four). An understanding of the distribution of LD regions is pivotal to developing rational approaches to the design and analysis of modern association studies. One of the most exciting developments recently is the capacity to undertake whole-genome scans based on indirect association rather than on linkage analysis[98]. Such scans are in part responsible for the striking recent progress that has been made in detecting genetic associations with complex diseases[126;127]: 'in the past three years genome–wide association studies (GWAS) .... have reproducibly identified hundreds of associations of common genetic variants with over 80 diseases and traits (www.genome.gov/gwastudies)'[128]. However, there are still many challenges to be met[25;99], as discussed in later chapters.

Genetic association studies aim to find correlations of differences in disease frequencies between groups (or in trait levels for continuously varying characters) with differences in their allele, or genotype, frequencies at a SNP. Thus, the frequencies of the two variant forms (alleles) of a SNP are of primary interest for identifying genes influencing disease. The simplest study design for assessment of genotype-phenotype correlations is the traditional *case-control* approach. However, this design carries the strong assumption that any observed differences in allele frequencies actually relate to the outcome measured; that is, there are no unobserved *confounding* influences, either directly attributable to the causal marker or through proximal association with it. Unfortunately, allele frequencies are known to vary widely within and between populations, irrespective of disease status. These confounding differences in allele frequency occur because each population is a product of its unique genetic and social history, and thus ancestral patterns of geographic migration, mating practices, reproductive expansions and bottlenecks and stochastic variation all yield allele frequency differences among individuals, yet none is necessarily related to any particular disease. These population frequency differences occur broadly throughout the genome and within many genes of known medical relevance. Consequently, the assumption of no confounding influences in genetic applications of the case-control design may be violated a priori for reasons that are at least partially outside the control of the investigator.

When cases and controls have different allele frequencies because of background population differences unrelated to outcome status, a study is said to suffer from *population stratification*. This is a potential problem for association studies using unrelated cases and controls as it can mimic the signal of association and lead to false positive or false negative results[95;100;101], especially when dealing with apparently ethnically homogeneous populations (see Chapter Four). This has been touted as one explanation for the repeated failure to replicate positive findings in genetic epidemiology[102;103] and remains the subject of an important ongoing debate[101-105]. The effects of population structure on association outcomes increase when attempting to detect small aetiological effects in studies with large sample sizes[101]— this is an important and topical issue for large national cohort and case-control initiatives of the type exemplified by UK Biobank[142] and the Wellcome Trust Case Control Consortium[143] (see Chapters Four and Six).

All approaches to the correction for population substructure demand a proper understanding of both genetics and epidemiology. Strategies might include: (1) family-based comparisons, such as sibling controls or case–parent triad designs, using the **transmission disequilibrium test** (TDT) or one of its variants[102;106;107]; (2) genetic markers (unlinked to a candidate gene) used to estimate the extent of bias induced by the stratification and subsequent correction using **genomic control**[101;108]; (3) **latent class modelling** based on a panel of markers that attempt to resolve the study population into a number of ethnically homogeneous subgroups, within which serious ethnic stratification is likely to be less problematic[109]; and (4) the use of sound epidemiological principles such as adjusting for, or stratifying by, *observed* ethnic group or place of ancestral origin. Strategy 4 necessitates availability of data on ethnic origin, ideally tracing back to grandparents[102]. There is a recognised need for a population genetics or genetic epidemiological study identifying the true extent of ethnic stratification within the indigenous (European origin) population of the United Kingdom.

Gene expression and gene product function

This book concentrates on the identification of genes in genomic DNA that may be implicated in the aetiology of complex diseases. However, this goes only part of the way towards fully understanding the biological pathways that lead to disease. There is a large and growing body of literature available about gene expression, gene product function, and the role of DNA, RNA and proteins in the living environment of an integrated organism, involving expert research across many fields. The central issues of these studies are quite different to the primary focus of this book, and although touched upon in Figure 1.1 and in Chapter Four, it is beyond the scope of this book to address these topics in detail. Readers interesting in more detail may find the following references of interest[144-146].

Genetic epidemiology in the future

For reasons based principally on considerations of statistical power and the ease of obtaining large samples, genetic epidemiology is increasingly moving away from linkage studies based on multiple-case families to allelic association studies based on unrelated individuals[19;25] (see Chapter Four).

One of the profound problems facing mainstream epidemiology[112;113] is that small aetiological effects of interest are being obscured by strong, unobserved covariates. In this context, it is relevant to note that the distribution of alleles at any given locus tends to be correlated neither with environmental exposures nor with the distribution of alleles at other loci – except for those few that are in tight LD[147]. Residual confounding can be largely circumvented when the biology underpinning genetic epidemiology is used to study the effect of key environmental determinants on diseases of public health. This approach is based on what is often called **Mendelian randomisation**[114-118; 148] (see Chapter Seven).

Studies involving at least 5,000 cases are now considered an essential element of the biomedical research infrastructure. These studies require huge national and international investment, resulting in often heated scientific debate – especially regarding study design. Even among the authors of this book, there is debate about key issues, including the role of large national cohort studies such as UK Biobank[116;119]. This debate is important and is a topic of discussion in Chapter Six.

Acknowledgments

P.R. Burton and M.D. Tobin are the joint first authors of the chapter and the order of their names is arbitrary. M.D. Tobin has been funded by UK MRC Fellowships G106/1008 and G0501942. The methodological research and educational programme in genomic epidemiology at the University of Leicester is supported by the programmes of: P³G (the Public Population Project in Genomics) funded by Genome Canada and Genome Quebec; PHOEBE (Promoting Harmonization of Epidemiological Biobanks in Europe) funded by the European Union under the Framework 6 programme; MRC Cooperative Grant G9806740; Programme Grant 00\3209 from the National Health and Medical Research Council (NHMRC) of Australia; and by Leverhulme Research Interchange Grant F/07134/K. J.L. Hopper is an Australian NHMRC Senior Principal Research Fellow. He is supported by Fellowship Grant 299955, and is a group leader of the Victorian Breast Cancer Research Consortium. Any views expressed are those of the authors and do not necessarily represent the views of the funding bodies.

References

1. Last JA, *Dictionary of Epidemiology*. New York: Oxford University Press, 2001.

2. Neel JV, Schull WJ, *Human Heredity*. Chicago, IL: Chicago University Press, 1954, 283–306.

3. Morton NE, Chung CS, *Genetic Epidemiology*. New York: Academic Press, 1978.

4. King MC, Lee GM, Spinner NB, *et al.*, Genetic Epidemiology. *Annual Review of Public Health*, 1984, 5, 1-52.

5. Morton NE, *Outline of Genetic Epidemiology*. London: Karger, 1982.

6. Roberts DF, A definition of genetic epidemiology. In Chakraborty R, Szathmary EJE, eds. *Diseases of Complex Etiology in Small Populations: Ethnic Differences and Research Approaches*. New York: Alan R Liss, 1985, 9–20.

7. Hopper JL, The epidemiology of genetic epidemiology. *Acta Geneticae Medicae at Gemellologiae*, 1992, 41, 261-73.

8. Mendel JG, The origins of genetics: a Mendel source book (translation). In Stern C, Sherwood E, eds. San Francisco: Freeman, 1966, 1–48.

9. Galton F, Hereditary talent and character. *MacMillan's Magazine*, 1865, 12, 157-66.

10. Fisher RA, The correlation between relatives on the supposition of Mendelian inheritance. *Transactions of the Royal Society of Edinburgh*, 1918, 52, 399-433.

11. Wijsman EM, Mendel's laws. In Elston R, Olsen J, Palmer L, eds. *Biostatistical Genetics and Genetic Epidemiology*. Chichester: Wiley, 2002, 527-9.

12. Botstein D, Risch N, Discovering genotypes underlying human phenotypes: past successes for Mendelian disease, future approaches for complex disease. *Nature Genetics*, 2003, 33 Suppl, 228-37

13. Palmer LJ, Complex diseases. In Elston R, Olsen J, Palmer L, eds. *Biostatistical Genetics and Genetic Epidemiology*. Chichester: Wiley, 2002, 141-3.

14. Risch NJ, Linkage strategies for genetically complex traits II. The power of affected relative pairs. *American Journal of Human Genetics*, 1990, 46, 229-41.

15. Lander ES, Kruglyak L. Genetic dissection of complex traits: guidelines for interpreting and reporting linkage results. *Nature Genetics*, 1995, 11, 241-7.

16. Todd JA, Interpretation of results from genetic studies of multifactorial diseases. *Lancet*, 1999, 354, 15-6.

17. Risch NJ, Searching for genetic determinants in the new millennium. *Nature*, 2000, 405, 847-56.

18. Colhoun HM, McKeigue PM, Davey Smith G, Problems of reporting genetic associations with complex outcomes. *Lancet*, 2003, 361, 865-72.

19. Zondervan KT, Cardon LR, The complex interplay among factors that influence allelic association. *Nature Reviews Genetics*, 2004, 5, 89-101.

20. Elston RC, The genetic dissection of multifactorial traits. *Clinical and Experimental Allergy*, 1995, 2, 103-6.

21. Elston R, Olsen J, Palmer L, *Biostatistical genetics and Genetic Epidemiology. Wiley Reference Series in Biostatistics*. Chichester: Wiley, 2002.

22. Strachan T, Read AP, *Human Molecular Genetics 3*. Oxford: Garland Science Publishers, 2003.

23. Lander ES, Linton LM, Birren B, *et al.*, Initial sequencing and analysis of the human genome. *Nature*, 2001, 409, 860-921.

24. Venter JC, Adams MD, Myers EW, *et al.*, The sequence of the human genome. *Science*, 2001, 291, 1304-51.

25. Carlson CS, Eberle MA, Kruglyak L, *et al.*, Mapping complex disease loci in whole-genome association studies. *Nature*, 2004, 429, 446-52.

26. International Human Genome Sequencing Consortium, Finishing the euchromatic sequence of the human genome. *Nature*, 2004, 431, 931-45.

27. Sham P. *Statistics in Human Genetics*. London: Arnold, 1998.

28. Balding DJ, Bishop M, Cannings C, *Handbook of Statistical Genetics*. Chichester: Wiley, 2003.

29. Burton PR, Tobin MD, Epidemiology and Genetic Epidemiology. In Balding DJ, Bishop M, Cannings C, eds. *Handbook of Statistical Genetics*, Chichester: Wiley, 2003.

30. Risch NJ, Linkage strategies for genetically complex traits I. Multilocus models. *American Journal of Human Genetics*, 1990, 46, 222-8.

31. Kopciuk KA, Bull SB, Risk Ratios. In Elston R, Olsen J, Palmer L, eds. *Biostatistical Genetics and Genetic Epidemiology*. Chichester: Wiley, 2002, 687-91.

32. Rothman K, Greenland S, Measures of Disease Frequency. In Rothman K, Greenland S, eds. *Modern Epidemiology. Second Edition*. Philadelphia: Lippincott-Raven, 1998, 29-46.

33. Rothman K, Greenland S, Types of Epidemiological Studies. In Rothman K, Greenland S, eds. *Modern Epidemiology. Second Edition*. Philadelphia: Lippincott-Raven, 1998, 67-78.

34. Guo S-W, Inflation of sibling recurrence-risk ratio, due to ascertainment bias and/or overreporting. *American Journal of Human Genetics*, 1998, 63, 252-8.

35. Weinberg W, Mathematische grundlagen der probandenmethode. *Zeitschrift fur Induktive Abstammungs un Vererbungslehre*, 1928, 48, 179-228.

36. Fisher RA, The effect of methods of ascertainment upon the estimation of frequencies. *Annals of Eugenics*, 1934, 6, 13-25.

37. Morton NE, Genetic tests under incomplete ascertainment. *American Journal of Human Genetics*, 1959, 11, 1-16.

38. Elston RC, Sobel E, Sampling considerations in the gathering and analysis of pedigree data. *American Journal of Human Genetics*, 1979, 31, 62-9.

39. Ewens WJ, Shute NC, The limits of ascertainment. *Annals of Human Genetics*, 1986, 50, 399-402.

40. Kraft P, Thomas DC, Bias and efficiency in family-based gene-characterisation studies: conditional, prospective, retrospective amd joint likelihoods. *American Journal of Human Genetics*, 2000, 66, 1119-31.

41. Hodge SE. Ascertainment. In Elston R, Olsen J, Palmer L, eds. *Biostatistical Genetics and Genetic Epidemiology*. Chichester: Wiley, 2002, 20-8.

42. Burton PR, Palmer LJ, Jacobs K, *et al.,* Ascertainment adjustment: where does it take us? *American Journal of Human Genetics*, 2000, 67, 1505-14.

43. Burton PR, Erratum: Ascertainment adjustment: where does it take us? *American Journal of Human Genetics*, 2001, 69, 692.

44. Burton PR, Correcting for non-random ascertainment in generalized linear mixed models (GLMMs) fitted using Gibbs sampling. *Genetic Epidemiology*, 2003, 24, 24-35.

45. Risch NJ, The genetic epidemiology of cancer: interpreting family and twin studies and their implications for molecular genetic approaches. *Cancer Epidemiology, Biomarkers & Prevention*, 2001, 10, 733-41.

46. Cookson W, Palmer L, Investigating the asthma phenotype. *Clinical and Experimental Allergy*, 1998, 28, 88-9.

47. Goldgar DE, Easton DF, Cannon-Albright LA, *et al.*, Systematic population-based assessment of cancer risk in first-degree relatives of cancer probands . *J Natl Cancer Inst*, 1994, 86, 1600-8.

48. Galton F, Typical laws of heredity. *Proceedings of the Royal Institution*, 1877, 8, 282-301.

49. Galton F, Family likeness in stature. *Proceedings of the Royal Society*, 1886, 40, 42-73.

50. Pearson K, Mathematical contributions to the theory of evolution - III. Regression, heredity and panmixia. *Philosophical Transactions of the Royal Society, Series A*, 1896, 187, 253-318.

51. Burton PR, Gurrin L, Sly P, Extending the simple linear regression model to account for correlated responses: An introduction to generalized estimating equations and multi-level mixed modelling. *Statistics in Medicine*, 1998, 17, 1261-91.

52. Goldstein H, *Multilevel Models in Educational and Social Research*. London: Charles Griffin and Company Ltd, 1987.

53. Zeger SL, Liang KY, An overview of methods for the analysis of longitudinal data. *Statistics in Medicine*, 1992, 11, 1825-39.

54. Neale MC, Cardon LR, Methodology for Genetic Studies of Twins and Families. Boston: Kluwer, 1992.

55. Breslow NE, Clayton DG, Approximate inference in generalized linear mixed models. *Journal of the Americal Statistical Association*, 1993, 88, 9-25.

56. Burton PR, Tiller KJ, Gurrin LC, *et al.*, Genetic variance components analysis for binary phenotypes using generalized linear mixed models (GLMMs) and Gibbs sampling. *Genetic Epidemiology*, 1999, 17, 118-40.

57. Armitage P, Berry G, and Matthews JNS, *Statistical Methods in Medical Research. (4th edition)*. Oxford: Blackwell Scientific Publications, 2002.

58. Peto J, Genetic predisposition to cancer. In Cairns J, Lyon JL, Skolnick M, eds. *Banbury Report 4: Cancer incidence in defined populations*. Cold Spring Harbour Laboratory, 1980, 203-13.

59. Hopper JL, Carlin JC, Familial aggregation of a disease consequent upon correlation between relatives in a risk factor measured on a continuous scale. *American Journal of Epidemiology*, 1992, 136, 1138-47.

60. Hopper JL, Variance components for statistical genetics: applications in medical research to characteristics related to human disease and health. *Statistical Methods in Medical Research*, 1993, 2, 199-223.

61. Khoury MJ, Beaty TH, Cohen BH, *Fundamentals of Genetic Epidemiology*. Oxford: Oxford University Press, 1993.

62. Hopper JL, Mathews JD, Extensions to multivariate normal models for pedigree analysis. *Annals of Human Genetics*, 1982, 46, 373–83.

63. Hopper JL, Visscher PM, Variance Component Analysis. In Elston R, Olsen J, Palmer L, eds. *Biostatistical Genetics and Genetic Epidemiology*. Chichester: Wiley, 2002, 778–88.

64. Jinks JL, Fulker DW, Comparison of the biometrical, genetical, MAVA, and classical approaches to the analysis of human behavior. *Psychological Bulletin*, 1970, 73, 5, 311–349.

65. Duffy DL, Martin NG, Inferring the direction of causality in cross-sectional twin data: theoretical and empirical considerations. *Genetic Epidemiology*, 1994, 11, 6, 483–502.

66. Neale MC, Twin analysis. In Elston R, Olsen J, Palmer L, eds. *Biostatistical Genetics and Genetic Epidemiology*. Chichester: Wiley, 2002, 743–56.

67. Hopper JL, Heritability. In Elston R, Olsen J, Palmer L, eds. *Biostatistical Genetics and Genetic Epidemiology*. Chichester: Wiley, 2002, 371–2.

68. Fisher RA. Limits to intensive production in animals. *British Agricultural Bulletin*, 1951, 4, 217–8.

69. Falconer DS, The inheritance of liability to certain disease, estimated from the incidence among relatives. *Annals of Human Genetics*, 1965, 29, 51–71.

70. Hopper JL, Hannah MC, Mathews JD, Genetic Analysis Workshop II. Pedigree analysis of a binary trait without assuming a liability. *Genetic Epidemiology*, 1984, 1, 2, 183–8.

71. Lichtenstein P, Holm NV, Verkasalo PK, *et al.*, Environmental and heritable factors in the causation of cancer – analyses of cohorts and twins from Sweden, Denmark and Finland. *New England Journal of Medicine*, 2000, 343, 78–85.

72. Hoover RN, Cancer – nature, nurture or both. *New England Journal of Medicine*, 2000, 343, 135–6.

73. Spector N, Shapiro BL, Peto R, *et al.*, Cancer, genes and environment (correspondence). *New England Journal of Medicine*, 2000, 343, 1494–6.

74. Hopper JL, Macaskill G, Powles JG, *et al.*, Pedigree analysis of blood pressure in subjects from rural Greece and relatives who migrated to Melbourne, Australia. *Genetic Epidemiology*, 1992, 9, 225–38.

75. Majumder PP, Segregation analysis, Classical. In Elston R, Olsen J, Palmer L, eds. *Biostatistical Genetics and Genetic Epidemiology*. Chichester: Wiley, 2002, 693–6.

76. Blangero J. Segregation Analysis, Complex. In Elston R, Olsen J, Palmer L, eds. *Biostatistical Genetics and Genetic Epidemiology*. Chichester: Wiley, 2002, 696–708.

77. Palmer LJ, Cookson WO, James AL, *et al.*, Gibbs sampling –based segregation analysis of asthma–associated quantitative traits in a population based sample of nuclear families. *Genetic Epidemiology*, 2001, 20, 356–72.

78. Terwilliger JD, Linkage analysis model based. In Elston R, Olsen J, Palmer L, eds. *Biostatistical Genetics and Genetic Epidemiology*. Chichester: Wiley, 2002, 448-60.

79. Elston RC. Segregation analysis. *Advanced Human Genetics*, 1981, 11, 372-3.

80. Cui J, Antoniou AC, Dite GS, *et al.,* After BRCA1 and BRCA1 - what next? Multifactorial analyses of three-generational, population-based Australian female breast cancer families. *American Journal of Human Genetics*, 2001, 68, 420-31.

81. Weiss ST, Raby BA, Asthma Genetics 2003. *Human Molecular Genetics Advance Access*, 2004, 13, 83R-9R.

82. Mathew CG, Lewis CM, Genetics of Inflammatory Bowel Disease: Progress and Prospects. *Human Molecular Genetics*, 2004, 13, 161R-8R.

83. Thompson EA, Linkage analysis. In Balding DJ, Bishop M, Cannings C, eds. *Handbook of Statistical Genetics*. Chichester: Wiley, 2001, 541-63.

84. Holmans P, Non-parametric linkage. In Balding DJ, Bishop M, Cannings C, eds. *Handbook of Statistical Genetics*. Chichester: Wiley, 2001, 487-505.

85. Olson JM, Linkage analysis model-based. In Elston R, Olsen J, Palmer L, eds. *Biostatistical Genetics and Genetic Epidemiology*. Chichester: Wiley, 2002, 461-72.

86. Fishel R, Lescoe MK, Rao MR, *et al.,* The human mutator gene homolog *MSH2* and its association with hereditary nonpolyposis colon cancer. *Cell*, 1993, 75, 1027-38.

87. Kolodner RD, Hall NR, Lipford J, *et al.,* Structure of the human MSH2 locus and analysis of two Muir-Torre kindreds for msh2 mutations. *Genomics*, 1994, 24, 516-26.

88. Kolodner RD, Hall NR, Lipford J, *et al.,* Structure of the human MLH1 locus and analysis of a large hereditary nonpolyposis colorectal carcinoma kindred for mlh1 mutations. *Cancer Research*, 1995, 55, 242-8.

89. Lynch HT, Lynch J, Lynch Syndrome: Genetics, Natural History, Genetic Counseling, and Prevention. *Journal of Clinical Oncology*, 2000, 18, 19s-31s.

90. Miki Y, Swensen J, Shattuck-Eidens D, *et al.,* A strong candidate for the breast and ovarian cancer susceptibility gene BRCA1. *Science*, 1994, 266, 66-71.

91. Wooster R, Bignell G, Lancaster J, *et al.,* Identification of the breast cancer susceptibility gene BRCA2. *Nature*, 1995, 378, 789-92.

92. Breslow NE, Day NE. Statistical Methods in Cancer Research. Volume 1: The analysis of case-control studies. Lyon: International Agency for research on Cancer, 1980.

93. Breslow NE, Day NE. Statistical Methods in Cancer Research. Volume 2: The design and analysis of cohort studies. Lyon: International Agency for Research on Cancer, 1987.

94. Scurrah KJ, Palmer LJ, Burton PR, Variance components analysis for pedigree-based censored survival data using generalized linear mixed models (GLMMs) and Gibbs sampling in BUGS. *Genetic Epidemiology*, 2000, 19, 127-48.

95. Clayton DG, Population association. In Balding DJ, Bishop M, Cannings C, eds. *Handbook of Statistical Genetics*. Chichester: Wiley, 2001, 519-40.

96. Chakravarti A. Linkage disequilibrium. In Elston R, Olsen J, Palmer L, eds. *Biostatistical Genetics and Genetic Epidemiology*. Chichester: Wiley, 2002, 472-5.

97. International HapMap Consortium. The International HapMap Project. *Nature*, 2003, 426, 789-96.

98. Arking DE, Pfeufer A, Post W, *et al.*, A common genetic variant in the NOS1 regulator NOS1AP modulates cardiac repolarization. *Nature Genetics*, 2006, 38, 644-51.

99. Wang H, Thomas DC, Pe'er I, *et al.*, Optimal Two-Stage Genotyping Designs for Genome-Wide Association Scans. *Genetic Epidemiology*, 2006, 30, 356–368.

100. Schaid DJ, Disease Marker Association. In Elston R, Olsen J, Palmer L, eds. *Biostatistical Genetics and Genetic Epidemiology*. Chichester: Wiley, 2002, 206-17.

101. Marchini J, Cardon LC, Phillips MS *et al.*, The effects of human population structure on large genetic association studies. *Nature Genetics*, 2004, 36, 512-7.

102. Thomas DC, Witte JS, Point: Population stratification: a problem for case-control studies of candidate-gene associations. *Cancer Epidemiology Biomarkers and Prevention*, 2002, 11, 505-12.

103. Cardon LR, Palmer LJ, Population stratification and spurious allelic association. *Lancet*, 2003, 361, 598-604.

104. Wacholder S, Rothman N, Caporaso N, Counterpoint: Bias from population stratification is not a major threat to the validity of conclusions from epidemiological studies of common polymorphisms and cancer. *Cancer Epidemiology Biomarkers and Prevention*, 2002, 11, 513-20.

105. Freedman LF , Reich D, Penney K, *et al.*, Assessing the impact of population stratification on genetic association studies. *Nature Genetics*, 2004, 36, 388 – 393.

106. Spielman RS, McGinnis RE, Ewens WJ, Transmission test for linkage disequilibrium: the insulin gene region and insulin-dependant diabetes mellitus (IDDM). *American Journal of Human Genetics*, 1993, 52, 506-16.

107. Ewens WJ, Spielman RS, The transmission/ disequilibrium test: history, subdivision and admixture. *American Journal of Human Genetics*, 1995, 57, 455-64.

108. Devlin B, Roeder K, Genomic control for association studies. *Biometrics*, 1999, 55, 997-1004.

109. Pritchard J, Stephens M, Donnelly P, Inference of population structure using multilocus genotype data. *Genetics*, 2000, 155, 945-59.

110. Terwilliger JD, Weiss KM, Linkage disequilibrium mapping of complex disease: fantasy or reality? *Current Opinion in Biotechnology*, 1998, 9, 578-94.

111. Hopper JL, Commentary: Case-control-family designs: a paradigm for future epidemiology research? *International Journal of Epidemiology*, 2003, 32, 48-50.

112. Taubes G. Epidemiology faces its limits. *Science*, 1995, 269, 164-9.

113. Davey Smith G, Ebrahim S, Epidemiology - is it time to call it a day? *International Journal of Epidemiology*, 2001, 30, 1-11.

114. Davey Smith G, Ebrahim S, 'Mendelian randomization': can genetic epidemiology contribute to understanding environmental determinants of disease? *International Journal of Epidemiology*, 2003, 32, 1-22.

115. Davey Smith G, Ebrahim S, Mendelian randomisation: prospects, potentials and limitations. *International Journal of Epidemiology*, 2004, 33, 30-42.

116. Clayton DG, McKeigue PM, Epidemiological methods for studying genes and environmental factors in complex diseases. *Lancet*, 2001, 358, 1356-60.

117. Tobin MD, Minelli C, Burtin PR, *et al.,* The development of Mendelian randomisation: from hypothesis testing to "Mendelian deconfounding". *International Journal of Epidemiology*, 2004, 33, 26-9.

118. Minelli C, Thompson JR, Tobin MD, *et al.,* An integrated approach to the meta-analysis of genetic association studies using Mendelian randomisation. *Americal Journal of Epidemiology*, 2004, 160, 445-52.

119. Burton PR, McCarthy M, Elliott P, Study of genes and environmental factors in complex diseases (comment). *Lancet*, 2002, 359, 1155-6.

120. Wright S, Correlation and causation. *Journal of Agricultural Research*, 1921, 20, 557-85.

121. Neale MC, Boker SM, Xie G, *et al., Mx: Statistical Modeling.* Virginia, USA: Richmond, 2002.

122. Lange K, Boehnke M, Weeks D, *Programs for Pedigree Analysis.* Los Angeles: Department of Biomathematics, UCLA, 1987.

123. Rasbash J, Browne W, Goldstein H, *et al., A User's Guide to MLwiN.* London: Institute of Education, 1999.

124. Spiegelhalter D, Thomas A, Best N, *WinBUGS Version 1.3 - User Manual.* Cambridge: MRC Biostatistics Unit, 2000.

125. Gauderman WJ, Thomas DC, Censored survival models for genetic epidemiology: a Gibbs sampling approach. *Genetic Epidemiology*, 1994, 11, 171-88.

126. Manolio TA, Brooks LD, and Collins FS, A HapMap harvest of insights into the genetics of common disease. *The Journal of Clinical Investigation*, 2008, 118, 1590-605.

127.　　Burton PR, Hansell AL, Fortier I, *et al.* Size matters: just how big is BIG? Quantifying realistic sample size requirements for human genome epidemiology. *Int J Epidemiol*, 2009, 38 (1): 263-73.

128.　　Hindorff LA, Sethupathy P, Junkins HA, Ramos EM, Mehta JP, Collins FS, *et al.* Potential etiologic and functional implications of genome-wide association loci for human diseases and traits. *Proceedings of the National Academy of Sciences*, 2009, 106 (23): 9362-67.

129.　　Burton PR, Tobin MD, Hopper JL, Key concepts in genetic epidemiology. *Lancet*, 2005, 366, 9489, 941-51.

130.　　Elston R, Linkage and association to genetic markers. *Experimental and Clinical Immunogenetics*, 1995, 12, 3, 129-40.

131.　　Haseman JK, Elston RC, The investigation of linkage between a quantitative trait and a marker locus. *Behavior Genetics*, 1972, 2, 3-19.

132.　　Morton NE, Sequential tests for the detection of linkage. *American Journal of Human Genetics*, 1956, 7, 277-318.

133.　　Ott J, Estimation of the recombination fraction in human pedigrees: efficient computation of the likelihood for human linkage studies. *American Journal of Human Genetics*, 1974, 26, 5, 588-97.

134.　　Lathrop GM, Lalouel JM, Julier C, *et al.*, Strategies for multilocus linkage analysis in humans. *Proceedings for the National Academy of Sciences* USA, 1984, 81, 11, 3443-6.

135.　　Bovee D, Zhou Y, Haugen E *et al.*, Closing gaps in the human genome with fosmid resources generated from multiple individuals. *Nature Genetics*, 2008, 40, 1, 96-101.

136.　　Wellcome Trust Case Control Consortium, Genome-wide association study of 14,000 cases of seven common diseases and 3,000 shared controls. *Nature*, 2007, 447, 7145, 661-78.

137.　　Feuk L, Carson AR, Scherer SW, Structural variation in the human genome. *Nature Reviews Genetics*, 2006, 7, 2, 85-97.

138.　　Freeman JL, Perry GH, Feuk L *et al.*, Copy number variation: new insights in genome diversity. *Genome Research*, 2006, 16, 8, 949-61.

139.　　Hopper JL, Variance components for statistical genetics: applications in medical research to characteristics related to human diseases and health. *Statistical Methods in Medical Research*, 1993, 2, 199-223.

140.　　Khoury M, Beaty T, Cohen B, *Fundamentals of genetic epidemiology*. Oxford: Oxford University Press, 1993.

141.　　Palmer LJ, Cookson WOCM. Genomic approaches to understanding asthma. *Genome Research*, 2000, 10, 9, 1280-7.

142.　　Altmuller J, Palmer LJ, Fischer G, *et al.*, Genomewide scans of complex human diseases: true linkage is hard to find. *American Journal of Human Genetics*, 2001, 69, 5, 936-50.

143.   Palmer LJ, Cardon LR, Shaking the tree: mapping complex disease genes with linkage disequilibrium. *Lancet*, 2005, 366, 9492, 1223-34.

144.   Terwilliger J, Linkage Analysis, Model-based. In: Elston RC, Olson JM, Palmer LJ, eds. *Biostatistical Genetics and Genetic Epidemiology*, pp449. Chichester: John Wiley and Sons, 2002.

145.   Palmer LJ, UK Biobank: bank on it. *Lancet*, 2007, 369, 9578, 1980-2.

146.   Wellcome Trust Case Control Consortium, Genome-wide association study of 14,000 cases of seven common diseases and 3,000 shared controls. *Nature*, 2007, 447, 7145, 661-78.

147.   van't Veer LJ, Bernards R, Enabling personalized cancer medicine through analysis of gene-expression patterns. *Nature*, 2008, 452, 7187, 564-70.

148.   Sieberts SK, Schadt EE, Moving toward a system genetics view of disease. *Mammalian Genome*, 2007, 18, 6-7, 389-401.

149.   Hobert O, Gene regulation by transcription factors and microRNAs. *Science*, 2008, 319, 5871, 1785-6.

150.   Davey Smith G, Lawlor DA, Harbord R, *et al.*, Clustered environments and randomized genes: a fundamental distinction between conventional and genetic epidemiology. *PLoS Medicine*, 2007, 4, 12, e352.

151.   Ebrahim S, Davey Smith G, Mendelian randomization: can genetic epidemiology help redress the failures of observational epidemiology? *Human Genetics*, 2008, 123, 1, 15-33.

TWO

Genetic linkage studies

M. Dawn Teare, Jennifer H. Barrett

Summary

Genetic linkage analysis can be used to identify regions of the genome that contain genes that may predispose individuals to disease, by mapping genetic loci from observations of related individuals. Linkage analysis methods can be applied to both major gene disorders (parametric linkage) and complex diseases (model-free or non-parametric linkage). Evidence for linkage is most commonly expressed as a logarithm of the odds score. A framework for interpretation of these scores will be provided in this chapter, and the role of simulation in assessment of statistical significance and estimation of power will be discussed. Genetic and phenotypic heterogeneity can also affect the success of a study, and several methods exist to address such problems.

Introduction

This chapter will explain the principles of linkage analysis in the context of major gene disorders and consider methods more suited to complex diseases that do not require the specification of a disease model (model-free or non-parametric linkage). The power and interpretation of linkage studies and the choice of phenotype will also be considered.

Linkage and linkage disequilibrium are two key concepts in genetic epidemiology (see Chapter One). Two genetic loci are linked if they are transmitted together from parent to offspring more often than expected under independent inheritance. They are in linkage disequilibrium if, across the population as a whole, they are found together on the same haplotype more often than expected (see Chapter Three). In general, two loci in linkage disequilibrium will also be linked, but the reverse is not necessarily true. Linkage extends over much longer regions of the genome than does linkage disequilibrium. Two loci are linked if, during meiosis, recombination occurs between them with a probability of less than 50% (see Chapter One). By contrast, every time recombination occurs between the loci in the population, the linkage disequilibrium between them is weakened, and is maintained only if the two loci are very close together. Linkage analysis is often the first stage in the genetic investigation of a trait, as it can be used to identify broad genomic regions that might contain a disease gene, even in the absence of previous biologically driven hypotheses.

Parametric linkage analysis

Parametric or model-based linkage analysis is the analysis of the co-segregation of genetic loci in pedigrees. Loci that are close enough together on the same chromosome segregate together more often than do loci on different chromosomes. Loci on different chromosomes segregate together purely by chance. Each genotype for one genetic marker or locus is made up of two alleles, one inherited from each parent. Specific alleles are in gametic phase when they are co-inherited from the same parent – they were present together in the single transmitted gamete originating from that parent. The further apart two loci are on the same chromosome, the more likely it is that a recombination event at meiosis will break up the co-segregation. The main quantity of interest in parametric linkage analysis is the **recombination fraction** θ, the probability of recombination between two loci at meiosis. By genotyping genetic markers and studying their segregation through pedigrees, it is possible to infer their position relative to each other on the genome. This process can be done to map genetic markers or to map disease or trait loci. There are now many sets of linkage-mapping markers, in which the markers have been selected to be regularly spaced across the genome (for example, the Marshfield Clinic resource at www.marshfieldclinic. org/research/pages/index.aspx).

Example: Ehlers-Danlos disease

As an example, Figure 2.1 shows a pedigree segregating a form of the Ehlers-Danlos disease (EDS-VIII, Mendelian Inheritance in Man (MIM) ID 130080; www.ncbi.nlm.nih.gov/omim/). The reported linkage analysis of this pedigree[3] will be used to illustrate parametric linkage analysis. EDS-VIII is a very rare autosomal dominant disorder. Five generations were clinically examined in this family, comprising 72 individuals, and DNA samples were available for genetic analysis from 19 of them. Figure 2.1 shows only those parts of the pedigree segregating the disease (many unaffected individuals are therefore not shown). The figure also shows genotypes for 17 selected genetic markers spanning 30 centimorgans (cM) on chromosome 12. For example, individual six is homozygous for allele 1 (denoted 1 1) for marker *D12S352*, whereas no genotype (denoted – –) is available for *D12S356*. This 30 cM region contains many more markers than those indicated. The bold black vertical line indicates a haplotype that is shared between affected individuals. In the third generation, affected individuals have co-inherited the same haplotype at all 17 loci, except for individuals 17 and 7; for individual 17, a recombination has occurred at some stage between markers *D12S100* and *D12S1615*. In the fourth generation, although three affected individuals still share the same full haplotype, there has been one recombination in individual 3 and evidence of two ancestral recombinations in individual 18. Ancestral recombinations refer to recombinations that have occurred in ancestors that cannot be directly discerned through genotyping. However, all affected individuals have co-inherited the same segment of chromosome 12, which is about 7 cM long (flanked by markers *D12S314* and *D12S1695*). Figure 2.1 shows that all individuals who have inherited the haplotype 6-10-5-3-7-6-3 between markers *D12S99* and *D12S336* has EDS type VIII, whereas no unaffected people have inherited this haplotype. Therefore this region of chromosome 12 could contain the dominant gene causing the disease.

Figure 2.1: Genotypes and haplotypes for a family with EDS-VIII for markers from chromosome 12p13

A square indicates male; a circle indicates a female; filled shapes indicate affected individuals; open shapes indicate unaffected individuals. The allele for each of the 17 markers are shown vertically in the following order, and the position of each marker relative to the first marker, *D12S352*, is as follows: *D12S100* (3.3 cM), *D12S1615* (4.6 cM), *D12S1626* (7.1 cM), *D12S1652* (7.6 cM), *D12S314* (11.4 cM), *D12S99* (12.6 cM), *D12S356* (14.2 cM), *D12S374* (14.2 cM), *D12S1625* (16.4 cM), *GATA49D12* (17.7 cM), *GATA151HO* (17.7 cM), *D12S336* (19.0 cM), *D12S1695* (19.6 cM), *GATA167AO* (20.3 cM), *D12S89* (23.2 cM), *D12S364* (29.4 cM). Reproduced with permission of University of Chicago Press[3].

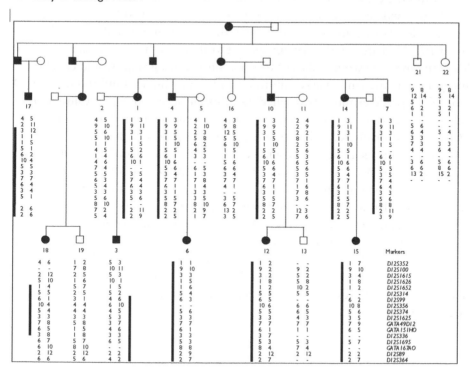

Logarithm of the odds scores

Linkage is usually reported as a **logarithm of the odds (LOD) score** (Box 2.1). This score was first proposed by Morton in 1955[5]. It is a function of the recombination fraction (θ) or chromosomal position, measured in cM. This means that the LOD score is different depending upon which value of θ is being considered. Large positive scores are evidence for linkage (or co-segregation), and negative scores are evidence against. To calculate a LOD score, a model for disease expression must be specified. This model includes the frequency of the disease allele and mode of inheritance (for example, dominant or recessive), marker allele frequencies, and a full marker map for each chromosome. The ultimate objective of the analysis is to estimate:

- the recombination fraction between individual markers and the disease locus (two–point); or
- the position of the disease locus relative to a fixed map of markers where the location of each marker is assumed to be known (multi–point).

The best (maximum likelihood) estimate of θ or position that maximises the LOD score function is the maximum LOD score. The higher the LOD score, the greater the evidence for linkage. Traditionally, a score of three was regarded as significant evidence of linkage. This is equivalent to $p = 0.0001$[6]. This seemingly stringent level of significance is because of the low prior probability of linkage to any particular marker and was originally set to allow for the sequential testing that Morton envisaged would follow. Morton assumed that groups would collaborate and genotype the same markers in more and more families until the total LOD score, for a predetermined θ, reached 3.0 (linkage accepted at that value of θ) or −2.0 (linkage rejected). However, the common practice now is to maximise the LOD score over the recombination fraction. This increases the power to detect linkage, and linkage is viewed as being excluded for all values of θ at which LOD is less than −2.0. More recent work shows that a LOD score of 3.0 is equivalent to a genome–wide significance level of about 0.09[7]. In this theoretical work, it was assumed that researchers could genotype markers at very high density over the whole genome (ten markers per cM). A higher threshold of at least 3.3 would be necessary to ensure that the genome–wide type 1 error (false positive) rate was in fact 0.05. Although the number of genetic markers used in a genome scan can be very large, once a certain density of markers is achieved, each new marker does not represent another independent statistical test and the threshold does not need to be increased.

Box 2.1: LOD scores and likelihood ratios

Results of genetic linkage studies are often reported in the form of LOD scores. These scores are actually based on likelihood ratios. The use of maximum likelihood in genetic linkage analysis was originally proposed in 1947[4]; its use became widespread once Morton[5] published his log-odds (LOD) tables, which enabled the sequential analysis of family-based linkage studies.

Maximum likelihood

Maximum likelihood provides a statistical framework to compare various hierarchical models and compute estimates of the various model parameters. The likelihood of the model, conditional on the data (represented as like[model]), is defined as the probability of the observations occurring, calculated according to the model. Hypotheses are tested by comparing two likelihoods (likelihood ratio test) – the likelihood of an alternative model versus the likelihood of the null (or reduced) model. Under the null model, twice the natural logarithm of the ratio of the likelihoods is distributed as a χ^2. Extreme values of the likelihood ratio test statistic are interpreted as evidence against the null hypothesis.

LOD scores

LOD score analysis is equivalent to likelihood ratio testing but, for historical reasons, instead of natural logarithms, logs to base 10 are used. In the linkage analysis framework, the only parameter of interest is the recombination fraction (θ) between marker and disease locus or the map position of the disease locus with respect to a fixed map of markers. The null hypothesis represents no linkage between disease and marker locus ($\theta = 0.5$), and the alternative hypothesis assumes linkage exists ($\theta < 0.5$). The LOD score function is then defined as:

$$LOD(\theta) = \log_{10} \left[\frac{Like(\theta)}{Like(\theta = \frac{1}{2})} \right]$$

The LOD score function is maximised with respect to θ – the recombination fraction in two-point analysis (a single marker and disease locus), or – map position in multi-point analysis (disease locus and at least two markers at fixed relative positions). The value of θ that gives the maximum LOD score is the maximum likelihood estimate of θ.

Heterogeneity LOD score

When linkage analysis is performed allowing for more than one disease locus, the LOD score is maximised with respect to two parameters, θ and α (the proportion of families linked to this locus). The heterogeneity LOD score is defined as:

LOD score for non-parametric sib pair linkage analysis

The classic likelihood ratio test statistic obtained from a non-parametric sibling pair linkage analysis is found by maximising the following ratio with respect to z_0 and z_1 (with $z_2 = 1 - z_0 - z_1$):

$$HLod(\alpha,\theta) = \log_{0}\left[\frac{Like(\alpha,\theta)}{Like(\alpha=1,\theta=\frac{1}{2})}\right]$$

This ratio can be converted into a LOD score for comparability with parametric analyses by dividing by 4.6 ($2 \times \log_e 10$), which changes the ratio to base 10 logarithms.

$$R\ (z_0,z_1) = 2\log_e\left[\frac{Like(z_0,z_1)}{Like(z_0=\frac{1}{4},z_1=\frac{1}{2})}\right]$$

Figure 2.2 is a plot of the LOD score function obtained when the EDS-VIII disease gene is assumed to be at one of a series of regularly spaced positions. The maximum score is obtained when the disease gene is placed close to marker *D12S356* (at 14.2 cM from *D12S352*). The LOD score decreases when moved away from this position, and at some points the score becomes very negative. Such large negative values are common in multi-point linkage analysis and this generally means that there is evidence that recombination(s) have arisen between marker(s) and the disease locus. For example, such a recombination has occurred between *D12S314* and *D12S99* for individual 3 in Figure 2.1. This individual has inherited allele 2 (*D12S314*) from the affected mother and must also have inherited the disease allele. This situation can only happen if there is recombination between the marker and disease. When the LOD score is calculated assuming the disease gene is coincident with marker *D12S314* (that is, these two locations are one and the same), one is assuming zero probability of recombination. So, in calculating the LOD score at this point, the recombination rate between the marker and disease locus is fixed to be zero. Joint consideration of data and model show this to be impossible or extremely unlikely, resulting in very strong evidence against linkage at that specific location.

Figure 2.2: Multipoint LOD score for EDS-VIII family by position (in cM) relative to marker closest to tip of chromosome 12 (D12S352 in this study)

The order and cumulative distance between markers were obtained from Marshfield Genetic Database and are presented in the same telomeric to centromeric order as in Figure 2.1, with positions relative to *D12S352* in parentheses: *D12S352* (0), *D12S100* (3.3 cM), *D12S1615* (4.6 cM), *D12S1626* (7.1 cM), *D12S1652* (7.6 cM), *D12S314* (11.4 cM), *D12S99* (12.6 cM), *D12S356* (14.2 cM), *D12S374* (14.2 cM), *D12S1625* (16.4 cM), *GATA49D12* (17.7 cM), *GATA151HO* (17.7 cM), *D12S336* (19.0 cM), *D12S1695* (19.6 cM), *GATA167AO* (20.3 cM), *D12S89* (23.2 cM), *D12S364* (29.4 cM). Reproduced with permission of University of Chicago Press[3].

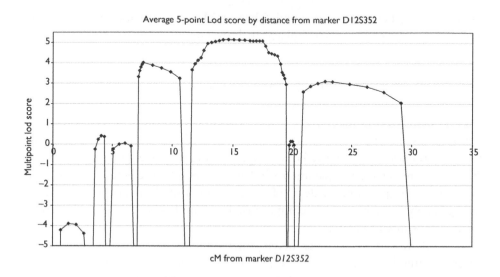

Specifying the genetic model

For any parametric linkage analysis, the genetic model for the disease of interest must be specified. For a simple Mendelian disease, this model amounts to mode of inheritance and frequency of disease allele. For some diseases, carrying the risk genotype does not always result in the individual being affected (**incomplete penetrance**). In more complex models, only a proportion of disease cases are due to a specific major gene, resulting in some risk of disease for individuals with any disease genotype (inclusion of a sporadic rate). Model parameters must be chosen before the linkage analysis. These model parameter estimates are preferably taken from population–based studies of the disease. Segregation analysis and estimation of familial relative risks can be used to ensure that appropriate models are used in the linkage analysis.

Genetic heterogeneity

The fact that the pattern of disease in families is consistent with a strong major gene component does not necessarily imply that only one gene is involved. There are many examples of diseases caused by inherited mutations in distinct genes. Some mutations give rise to the same disease but with a different mode of inheritance –

for example, Charcot–Marie–Tooth disease has autosomal recessive, dominant and X-linked forms, and mutations in up to ten genes are responsible for the different forms[8]. The EDS-VIII family illustrated in Figure 2.1 yielded strong evidence of a disease gene on chromosome 12, but, when four further smaller families were examined, two were not consistent with linkage to this region.

Heterogeneity LOD scores

Locus heterogeneity such as that with Charcot–Marie–Tooth disease can seriously affect the power of parametric linkage analysis. The most common solution is to assume that mutations in the disease genes will be so rare that each family will be linked to only one such gene. The genome scan is then done, maximising a heterogeneity LOD score (Box 2.1). At each genomic position, the heterogeneity LOD score is maximised with respect to another parameter α, the proportion of families linked to this locus. If the genetic component of a disease is due to a few major genes, then power to detect linkage is reduced, but it might still be possible to detect the locus in this way. For example, the breast cancer genes *BRCA1* and *BRCA2* were detected by parametric linkage analysis despite heterogeneity[9; 10]. If the genetic component is made up of a large number of distinct genes, parametric linkage analysis can be severely compromised and model-free alternatives become necessary, as discussed later.

Methods for reducing locus heterogeneity include limiting the analysis to strictly defined subtypes of disease (where there might be reason to suspect a stronger genetic component or where subtypes might themselves be diseases with distinct causes, each with a distinct genetic component) or targeting families in an isolated population where the number of original founder mutations could be low. Standard methods for accounting for heterogeneity assume that the genetic model for disease will be the same in linked and unlinked families. If genetic heterogeneity exists, then the estimates of model parameters from population genetics might no longer be appropriate when trying to identify individual loci contributing to the overall genetic component. It is therefore common for genome scans to be done for a range of parametric models allowing for heterogeneity. However, if the LOD score has been maximised over several models, then to maintain a low false positive rate the threshold (3.3) will need to be raised. The significance of the resulting maximum LOD score can be estimated by simulation.

Model-free (non-parametric) linkage analysis

For multi-factorial diseases, where several genes (and environmental factors) might contribute to disease risk, there is no clear mode of inheritance. Methods to investigate linkage have therefore been developed that do not require specification of a disease model. Such methods are referred to as **non-parametric** or **model-free**. The rationale is that, between affected relatives, excess sharing of haplotypes that are identical by descent (IBD) in the region of a disease-causing gene would be expected, irrespective of the mode of inheritance. Various methods test whether IBD sharing at a locus is greater than expected under the null hypothesis of no linkage.

Sibling pairs

The simplest approach is to study sibling pairs, both of whom are affected. At any locus, according to the null hypothesis of no linkage, the number of IBD alleles shared by a pair of siblings is none with probability 0.25, one with probability 0.5, or two with probability 0.25 (Box 2.2). If IBD sharing in the families is known, the observed proportions of pairs sharing no, one and two alleles at a candidate locus can be compared with these expectations. Linkage would be suggested if the pairs of siblings, both of whom are affected by a disease, share significantly more alleles IBD than expected by chance. The best test for linkage to use depends on the true mode of inheritance, but in a wide range of situations the most powerful test is the so-called mean test, in which the mean number of alleles shared IBD is compared with the expected value of one[11].

In practice, IBD sharing between a pair of siblings is rarely known with complete certainty because the parents may not have been genotyped and the markers might not be sufficiently polymorphic to distinguish between sharing IBD or identical by state (IBS) (Box 2.2). In such cases, the proportions of IBD sharing can only be estimated. A general algorithm for calculating these proportions considers all possible parental genotypes that are consistent with the data[12]. More recently, maximum likelihood methods have been used[13–17].

Other groups of relatives

Pairwise comparisons between relatives can easily be modified for types of relative pairs other than siblings. However, in studies that set out to examine affected sibling pairs, additional affected siblings are often recruited. Various methods have been proposed to extend the pairwise approach to sibships larger than two. Selecting one pair at random or using only independent pairs means discarding information, so using all possible pairs is preferred. However, should larger sibships be downweighted to account for non-independence between pairs with this approach? If so, how?[18;19] Weighting might improve power, but given that the type 1 error rate depends on factors such as the informativeness of the markers, it is recommended that significance levels be estimated by simulation[19;20], a point that will be expanded on below.

Alternative methods have been developed to analyse families with larger numbers of affected relatives of differing relationship, also based on the degree of IBD sharing. Each pedigree can be assigned a score that measures IBD sharing, and the test for linkage is based on comparing this score with the expected score according to the null hypothesis (combining over pedigrees). The score can be based on pairwise comparisons, but a more powerful alternative score has been

Box 2.2: Allele-sharing in sibling pairs

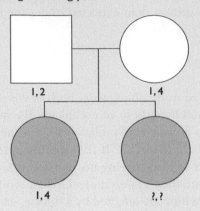

In this affected sibling pair the sister on the left has inherited allele 1 from her father and allele 4 from her mother. If the marker is unlinked to the disease, there are four equally likely combinations of alleles the second sister can inherit: (1,1), (1,4), (2,1) or (2,4), where the first number indicates the paternally inherited allele and the second number the maternally inherited allele. As illustrated in the table below, the numbers of alleles shared by the sisters that are IBD are 1, 2, 0 and 1, respectively. This leads to the IBD sharing probabilities of 0.25 (for sharing 0), 0.5 (for sharing 1) and 0.25 (for sharing 2) referred to in the text. IBD sharing must be distinguished from the numbers of alleles shared that are identical by state (IBS). When the second sister has genotype (2,1), both sisters have a type 1 allele; these alleles are IBS, but they are not IBD (assuming the parents are not inbred) because one is inherited from the father and one from the mother.

Genotype		Number of alleles shared	
Sibling 1	Sibling 2	IBD	IBS
1,4	1,1	1	1
	1,4	2	2
	2,1	0	1
	2,4	1	1

proposed[21] that increases sharply as the number of affected members sharing the same allele IBD increases. This score is used by the program Genehunter[22]. Provided that many similar families are studied, under the null hypothesis, the resulting non–parametric linkage test statistic is normally distributed with mean of zero and variance of one. In the absence of complete information, the score is replaced by its estimated value, leading to a conservative test. These methods have been modified to provide accurate likelihood–based tests[23], all implemented in the much faster program Allegro[24].

In linkage studies, genotyping is usually done at a set of linked markers (in some cases covering the whole genome). Here, IBD sharing can be estimated more accurately by multi-point analysis, by use of information from all markers on the chromosome. At any point along a chromosome, the pattern of inheritance within a pedigree can be described by an **inheritance vector.** This vector records, for each non-founding member of the family, whether they have inherited the grandpaternal or grandmaternal allele from each of their parents. The full inheritance vector might not be uniquely determined by the marker data, but its probability distribution, conditional on the marker data, can be calculated[17]. Calculation of the full multi-point IBD distribution for a pedigree is a non-trivial problem. Most available methods are based on algorithms that are limited either in the number of markers or in the complexity of the pedigrees that can be analysed. To cope with problems of large size in both dimensions, methods have been developed based on Markov chain Monte Carlo estimation[25]. Recently, whole-genome screens have been performed with several thousand SNPs[26; 27; 28], increasing the number of markers by an order of magnitude over previous methods. An analytical method based on gene flow trees has been developed to handle such data, implemented in the program Merlin[29]. One advantage of this approach is the considerable increase in information content compared with standard panels of microsatellite markers[27; 28] although, in principle, a denser set of microsatellites could be used to increase information. A further advantage is that SNP genotyping can be carried out with very high degrees of accuracy. Care needs to be taken that SNPs in linkage disequilibrium with each other are not included in the analysis, because this can lead to false positive results using available methods of linkage analysis (which assume linkage equilibrium between markers[27; 30]).

There have been corresponding methodological developments in quantitative trait linkage analysis. Haseman and Elston (1972)[12] suggested using sibling pairs to investigate linkage by regressing the squared difference in the siblings' trait values on the (estimated) proportion of alleles shared IBD. Two siblings that share more alleles IBD would be expected to have more similar trait values if the marker is linked to a gene influencing the trait. Consequently, in the presence of such linkage, there should be a negative relation between the squared trait differences and the estimated IBD sharing. More powerful variants of this method have since been developed that also incorporate information from the sum of the siblings' trait values, for example using the mean-corrected cross-product (**sibling covariance**) as the dependent variable[31] (Box 2.3). Variance components methods have been developed to analyse quantitative trait linkage in general pedigrees. These methods model the trait covariance between relatives, partitioning this value into components due to a specific chromosomal region (on the basis of estimated IBD sharing) and unlinked genes (on the basis of degree of kinship). These methods can now be undertaken with multi-point methods to estimate IBD sharing (for example with the program SOLAR[32]).

A large number of whole-genome screens in a wide range of complex diseases have now been done with model-free linkage analysis for both qualitative and quantitative traits. One example was an affected sibling pair study of type 1 diabetes[39], which successfully identified linkage to the human leukocyte antigen

Box 2.3: Quantitative trait linkage analysis using sibling pairs

Suppose we have a set of sibling pairs, and let the trait values for the jth sibling pair be x_{1j} and x_{2j}. In the original method proposed[9], the squared difference in trait values $(x_{1j} - x_{2j})^2$ is regressed on the number of alleles shared IBD. This dependent variable ignores the information in the *sum* of the siblings' trait values, which would also be related to the number of alleles shared IBD under the alternative hypothesis.

Combining the sum and the difference in trait values (corrected by the overall mean trait value μ), the following dependent variable is suggested:

$$((x_{1j} - \mu) + (x_{2j} - \mu))^2 - ((x_{1j} - \mu) - (x_{2j} - \mu))^2$$

which simplifies to give a multiple of the mean-corrected cross-product:

$$4(x_{1j} - \mu)(x_{2j} - \mu)$$

The expected value of the mean-corrected cross-product is the **sibling covariance**.

(HLA) region with a LOD score of more than 7. Many quantitative traits related to cardiovascular disease have been investigated, with some interesting results; for example, in a whole-genome screen of high-density lipoprotein cholesterol, evidence of linkage to a locus on chromosome 9p was identified[40]. A review of genome screens of complex diseases[41] showed that few studies published before 2001 were able to demonstrate significant linkage, according to the criteria of Lander and Kruglyak[7] described below. The completion of hundreds of family-based genome-wide scans for linkage to complex disease genes with little success in gene discovery, coupled with the availability of high-density SNP maps across the genome and decreasing genotyping costs, has shifted emphasis away from linkage analysis and microsatellite markers towards SNP genotyping and different analytical strategies based on allelic association (see Introduction and Chapters Three and Four).

There has also been further analytical development in the investigation of gene-environment and gene-gene interactions. The inclusion of a covariate in linkage analysis can be a powerful method of accounting for disease heterogeneity, and there are numerous examples in which the evidence for linkage has been enhanced by this approach[35; 36; 59]. This method allows the degree of IBD sharing to be dependent on a covariate such as sex or history of smoking[33; 34]. Similarly gene-gene interactions have been investigated, usually looking for interaction with established disease loci[37], but also using a systematic 'two-dimensional' linkage scan[38]. Such methods are contributing to addressing the expected complexity of disease risk, and are a promising way forward provided care is taken in the interpretation of results.

Issues of power and interpretation

A fundamental issue in understanding the results of a linkage analysis is the interpretation of statistical significance. Whenever statistical tests are performed, a balance must be struck between making claims of which many fail to be substantiated and adopting criteria so stringent that true findings are missed. For the parametric analysis of single gene disorders, it was suggested early that a threshold of 3.0 for the LOD score indicated a significant result at the genome-wide level. This approach has been instrumental in avoiding the reporting of large numbers of false-positive results but at the same time allowing linkage analyses of single-gene disorders to lead successfully to the identification and cloning of disease genes.

The threshold issue is more contentious with complex traits. In 1995, Lander and Kruglyak[7] made proposals that have proved highly influential. Assuming a dense map of fully informative markers, they used mathematical theory to derive the threshold required for a LOD score to achieve genome-wide significance of 5%. Because the LOD scores used in different approaches have slightly different properties, the thresholds vary slightly from method to method. For parametric linkage analysis, a threshold of 3.3 is necessary, whereas in an affected sibling pair study significant linkage needs a LOD score of 3.6 (or 4.0 if the so-called possible triangle constraints[16] are used). From a whole-genome scan, Lander and Kruglyak suggested that areas of suggestive linkage (evidence expected to occur once overall by chance) and nominal linkage ($p = 0.05$ from a single test without adjustment for multiple testing) should also be reported, although in the latter case no claims for linkage should be made.

The stringency of the criteria for genome-wide significance has been questioned, because they are based on the assumption of a dense marker map with no missing data. An alternative and flexible approach is to perform a simulation, which can take particular features of the study into account. Datasets can be simulated according to the null hypothesis of no linkage across the whole genome with the same family structures, marker map, allele frequencies and patterns of missing data as in the study itself. With advances in computing, simulation is becoming the standard method of assessment in large studies[40; 42-45]. This approach also has the advantage that the correct significance level can be identified for any method of analysis and is particularly valuable when interactions are considered.

The threshold for statistical significance from empirical simulation is likely to be lower than that from theoretical results as it is based on the specific features of a particular dataset; how much lower will depend on the features of the study. For a whole-genome scan of siblings with multiple sclerosis that used simulation[20], it was estimated that a LOD score of 3.2 would be achieved without linkage in only one in 20 studies – that is, a LOD score of 3.2 would be significant at the genome-wide level at 5% . Further investigation suggested that map density and the extent of missing data have a substantial effect on significance levels[46]. Even if no locus were to show significant evidence of linkage, a genome-wide study could contain independent peaks of linkage exceeding some lower threshold (for example, 2.0). In the locus counting approach, a series of such thresholds is considered, and the number of independent regions expected to exceed these thresholds under the null hypothesis of no linkage is estimated by simulation. This null distribution is then used to interpret the results of the genome screen, by determining whether more peaks than would be expected by chance were evident.

Considerations of genome-wide significance apply to whole-genome scans, but it can be argued that the situation is not so much different in candidate-gene linkage studies. Here, instead of whole-genome scanning, regions containing genes selected on biological grounds are investigated. In practice, because for most diseases a good case can be made for a very large number of candidates, the significance of results should not be interpreted very differently from those of genome-wide scans. Often numerous subgroup analyses are also undertaken, which can again inflate the false-positive rate if not interpreted correctly.

Simulation has an equally important role in study design. Genetic linkage studies can be expensive and investigators will not want to begin a study with low power. Power calculations by simulation will inform decisions about the number and type of families required and the necessary marker density. Generally, the more affected individuals in a pedigree, the more informative the family is. However, some familial configurations will be more informative than others. The most common difficulty is missing data – there might be little available information about older family members and not all members of the family will consent to providing DNA. Simulation allows investigators to estimate the power of the family collections available for analysis.

The frequency of many diseases varies widely between populations. This differential incidence can be due to variations in both environmental and genetic background. For example, the autosomal recessive Tay–Sachs disease is 100 times more common in Ashkenazi Jews than non-Jews[47], and site-specific cancer shows a very high degree of variation in incidence even within Europe[48]. Many forms of genetic differences have been identified between populations[49], and studies may need to consider these additional sources of heterogeneity and allow for them in the analysis if possible. Such population differences usually reduce statistical power. The limited success of linkage analysis for complex diseases so far is at least in part due to studies being too small to detect genes of modest effect. The interpretation of apparently negative findings depends crucially on power. The sample size necessary to detect linkage to genes with a genotype relative risk of less than two could be unachievable[50]. Genotype error also affects power[51]. With large pedigrees, genotype error is easy to detect because such errors often lead to Mendelian inconsistencies within the pedigree. However, where only affected sibling pairs are genotyped, with no other family data, incorrect genotypes will probably not be detected.

Choice of phenotype

Some traits or diseases have a clear phenotype definition. For simple Mendelian traits, it is straightforward to identify affected and unaffected individuals. Even in a disease such as cancer, once symptoms are experienced the diagnosis is based on pathological findings. However, other illnesses such as psychiatric disorders are more problematic because the diagnosis often depends on several distinct symptoms, and there is often disagreement as to what constitutes a definitive diagnosis[52]. The absence of a clear definition of phenotype will lead to uncertainty about the classification of affected and unaffected individuals and to potential inconsistency between studies. Sometimes, the use of a quantitative trait can circumvent this difficulty; for example, the number of distinct symptoms could be used as a measure of disease severity. Conversely, there may sometimes be good reason to transform a quantitative trait into a binary one. For example, an individual may be classed as obese if their body mass index is above a defined threshold and non-obese if it is below it. However, simplifying a quantitative trait to a binary phenotype can result in loss of power if an inappropriate threshold is used[53].

Genetic linkage studies are very rarely done with population-based family datasets. Usually some other selection criteria are applied to the phenotype before the families are selected. These criteria are often driven by the need to maximise power and to reduce heterogeneity. A disease is aetiologically heterogeneous if it can result from more than one distinct pathway. Families are usually selected because of segregation of the disease of interest and might be studied only if many members are affected. There might also be a focus on severely affected individuals such as those with early age at onset or those with other critical symptoms. Some diseases, such as Charcot-Marie-Tooth disease, might be classified into clear clinical subtypes. Sometimes diseases can be associated with other phenotypes, and families can be categorised as to whether or not the other phenotype is present – for example families with breast cancer with or without ovarian cancer within the pedigree. Eligibility criteria such as these can reduce heterogeneity, and it can be advantageous at the analysis stage if datasets can be split into meaningful subgroups. However, these sampling strategies can cause problems later when trying to interpret the linkage finding in terms of the general population. For example, if a study finds that in half of a selected number of families a disease is linked to a specific locus, these results may not necessarily predict the proportion of the disease due to this locus in the broader population.

If the phenotype of interest is a diagnosis requiring treatment or registration, the eligible families will often be ascertained via specialist clinics. In other cases, the phenotype itself might not be a treatable disease but a risk factor for disease. A good example of this is obesity. Obesity can be measured in different ways and therefore studies can be difficult to compare; there is also the additional problem of ascertainment. Most linkage studies of obesity have arisen through datasets designed to study other primary endpoints such as heart disease, osteoporosis and diabetes. There have been a large number of published linkage studies of obesity-related phenotypes[60; 61]. Many of these individually large studies have reported significant linkage, but few such findings have been replicated, indicating not only genetic heterogeneity and low power, but also the heterogeneity of study designs and choice of phenotype. It is only with the move to genome-wide association scans that real progress has begun to be made with complex phenotypes such as obesity.

One way of tackling replication of linkage results in complex diseases is through the meta-analysis of results from multiple studies[55;56]. However, meta-analysis works best when studies have been done under homogeneous conditions, when phenotypes have been measured with the same criteria and when statistical analyses have been similar. Datasets may need to be recoded before a meta-analysis is done. For complex phenotypes such as obesity, where ascertainment is so variable, collaborative analyses on raw data are essential.

Linkage analysis: what next?

A linkage analysis of the whole genome can identify regions that show evidence of containing a disease gene. In the study of Mendelian traits, crossover events often narrow down the region sufficiently to define a small interval of interest, and this has resulted in the mapping of over 2,000 new genes[62]. Linkage clearly remains the method of choice for mapping single-gene disorders. Linkage analysis of complex diseases has resolution to identify only large regions of interest (typically tens of cM). Location estimates indicated by the linkage peak are highly variable, and increasing the density of the marker map improves the resolution only somewhat [57]. Although a very strong candidate gene might exist within the linkage region, such regions often contain hundreds of genes, many of which are biologically plausible candidates. One way to narrow the region in studies of cancer is by examining the loss of heterozygosity in tumours[58]. When markers that are heterozygous in germline DNA exhibit loss of heterozygosity in tumour cells, this can indicate deletion of a region of the chromosome, and the pattern of such loss can be used to narrow down the location of a tumour suppressor gene. However, methods development in linkage analysis continues[63], and linkage analysis will probably remain useful for investigating specific, mono- or oligogenic forms of complex disease (for example the *BRCA1* mutation in breast cancer[64]). With an increasing understanding of disease pathogenesis and the concomitant better ability to define subphenotypes, as has happened in neuropsychiatric disease[65], linkage analysis will probably have an ongoing role to play in complex disease genetics. This is particularly so given the renewed interest in translating family history and gene-associated risk into clinical practice following successful gene discoveries arising from genome-wide association scans[66]. Current mapping approaches to gene discovery in complex disease are based on linkage disequilibrium, which extends over much smaller distances than linkage. These methods are the subject of Chapter Three. The current association-based paradigm for gene discovery in common human diseases is centred entirely on the common-disease common-variant hypothesis – that is, it assumes that we are looking for common variants of modest effect for each disease[54; 67]. The strategy, based on tagging SNPs and genome-wide association scans, has been very successful at finding such genes for many complex diseases (see Chapter Four). However, as gene mapping projects for complex human diseases turn their attention to rarer genes, which are much harder (and in some cases may be impossible) to detect using population-based association designs, it is likely that family-based studies and linkage analysis will once more become central to genetic epidemiology.

References

1. Burton PR, Tobin MD, Hopper JL, Key concepts in genetic epidemiology. *Lancet*, 2005; 366, 941–51.

2. Cordell HJ, Clayton DG, Genetic association studies. *Lancet*, 2005; 366, 9491, 1121-31.

3. Rahman N, Dunstan M, Teare MD *et al.,* Ehlers-Danlos syndrome with severe early-onset periodontal disease (EDS-VIII) is a distinct, heterogeneous disorder with one predisposition gene at chromosome 12p13. *American Journal of Human Genetics*, 2003; 73, 198–204.

4. Haldane JBS, Smith CAB, A new estimate of the linkage between the genes for colour-blindness and haemophilia in man. *Annals of Eugenics*, 1947; 14, 10–31.

5. Morton NE, Sequential tests for the detection of linkage. *American Journal of Human Genetics*, 1955; 7, 277–318.

6. Chotai J, On the LOD score method in linkage analysis. *Annals of Human Genetics*, 1984; 48, 359–78.

7. Lander ES, Kruglyak L, Genetic dissection of complex traits: guidelines for interpreting and reporting linkage results. *Nature Genetics*, 1995; 11, 241–47.

8. Berger P, Young P, Suter U, Molecular cell biology of Charcot-Marie-Tooth disease. *Neurogenetics*, 2002; 4, 1–15.

9. Hall JM, Lee MK, Newman B, *et al.,* Linkage of early-onset familial breast cancer to chromosome 17q21. *Science*, 1990; 250, 1684–89.

10. Wooster R, Bignell G, Lancaster J, *et al.,* Identification of the breast cancer susceptibility gene BRCA2. *Nature*, 1995; 378, 789–92.

11. Blackwelder WC, Elston RC, A comparison of sib-pair linkage tests for disease susceptibility loci. *Genetic Epidemiology*, 1985; 2, 85–97.

12. Hasemen JK, Elston RC, The investigation of linkage between a quantitative trait and a marker locus. *Behavior Genetics*, 1972; 2, 3–19.

13. Risch N, Genetics of IDDM: evidence for complex inheritance with HLA. *Genetic Epidemiology*, 1989; 6, 143–48.

14. Risch N, Linkage strategies for genetically complex traits. III. The effect of marker polymorphism on analysis of affected relative pairs. *American Journal of Human Genetics*, 1990; 46, 242–53.

15. Risch N, Linkage strategies for genetically complex traits. II. The power of affected relative pairs. *American Journal of Human Genetics*, 1990; 46, 229–41.

16. Holmans P, Asymptotic properties of affected–sib–pair linkage analysis. *American Journal of Human Genetics*, 1993; 52, 362–74.

17. Kruglyak L, Lander ES, Complete multipoint sib-pair analysis of qualitative and quantitative traits. *American Journal of Human Genetics*, 1995; 57, 439–54.

18. Suarez BK, Van Eerdewegh P, A comparison of three affected-sibpair scoring methods to detect HLA-linked disease susceptibility genes. *American Journal of Medical Genetics*, 1984; 18, 135–46.

19. Holmans P, Likelihood-ratio affected sib-pair tests applied to multiply affected sibships: issues of power and type I error rate. *Genetic Epidemiology* 2001; 20, 44–56.

20. Sawcer S, Jones HB, Judge D, *et al.,* Empirical genomewide significance levels established by whole genome simulations. *Genetic Epidemiology*, 1997; 14, 223–29.

21. Whittemore AS, Halpern J, A class of tests for linkage using affected pedigree members. *Biometric,s* 1994; 50, 118–27.

22. Kruglyak L, Daly MJ, Reeve-Daly MP, *et al.,* Parametric and nonparametric linkage analysis: a unified approach. *American Journal of Human Genetics*, 1996; 58, 1347–63.

23. Kong A, Cox NJ, Allele-sharing models: LOD scores and accurate linkage tests. *American Journal of Human Genetics*, 1997; 61, 1179–88.

24. Gudbjartsson DF, Jonasson K, Frigge ML, *et al.,* Allegro, a new computer program for multipoint linkage analysis. *Nature Genetics*, 2000; 25, 12–13.

25. Sobel E, Lange K, Descent graphs in pedigree analysis: applications to haplotyping, location scores, and marker-sharing statistics. *American Journal of Human Genetics*, 1996; 58, 1323–37.

26. John S, Shepard N, Lui G, *et al.,* Whole-genome scan, in a complex disease, using 11, 245 single nucleotide polymorphisms: comparison with microsatellites. *American Journal of Human Genetics*, 2004; 75, 54–64.

27. Schaid DJ, Guenther JC, Christensen GB, *et al.,* Comparison of microsatellites versus single-nucleotide polymorphisms in a genome linkage screen for prostate cancer-susceptibility loci. *American Journal of Human Genetics*, 2004; 75, 948-965.

28. Amos CI, Chen WV, Lee A, *et al.,* High density SNP analysis of 642 Caucasian families with rheumatoid arthritis identifies two new linkage regions on 11p12 and 2q33. *Genes and Immunity*, 2006; 7, 277-286.

29. Abecasis GR, Cherny SS, Cookson WO, *et al.,* Merlin: rapid analysis of dense genetic maps using sparse gene flow trees. *Nature Genetics*, 2002; 30, 97–101.

30. Huang Q, Shete S, Amos CI, Ignoring linkage disequilibrium among tight linked markers induces false-positive evidence of linkage for affected sib pair analysis. *American Journal of Human Genetics*, 2004; 75, 1106-1112

31. Elston RC, Buxbaum S, Jacobs KB, *et al.,* Haseman and Elston revisited. *Genetic Epidemiology*, 2000; 19, 1–17.

32. Almasy L, Blangero J, Multipoint quantitative-trait linkage analysis in general pedigrees. *American Journal of Human Genetics*, 1998; 62, 1198–211.

33. Devlin B, Jones BL, Bacanu SA, *et al.,* Mixture models for linkage analysis of affected sibling pairs and covariates. *Genetic Epidemiology*, 2002: 22, 52-65.

34. Holmans P, Detecting gene-gene interactions using affected sib pair analysis with covariates. *Human Heredity*, 2002; 53, 92-102.

35. Goddard KA, Witte JS, Suarez BK, *et al.,* Model-free linkage analysis with covariates confirms linkage of prostate cancer to chromosomes 1 and 4. *American Journal of Human Genetics*, 2001; 68, 1197-1206.

36. Olson JM, Goddard KA, Dudek DM, The amyloid precursor protein locus and very-late-onset Alzheimer disease. *American Journal of Human Genetics*, 2001; 69, 895-899.

37. John S, Amos C, Shephard N, *et al.,* Linkage analysis of rheumatoid arthritis in US and UK families reveals interactions between HLA-DRB1 and loci on chromosomes 6q and 16p. *Arthritis and Rheumatism*, 2006; 54, 1482-1490.

38. Bell JT, Wallace C, Dobson R, *et al.,* Two-dimensional genome-scan identifies novel epistatic loci for essential hypertension. *Human Molecular Genetics*, 2006; 15, 1365-1374.

39. Davies JL, Kawaguchi Y, Bennett ST, *et al.,* A genome-wide search for human type 1 diabetes susceptibility genes. *Nature*, 1994; 371, 130–136.

40. Arya R, Duggirala R, Almasy L, *et al.,* Linkage of high-density lipoprotein-cholesterol concentrations to a locus on chromosome 9p in Mexican Americans. *Nature Genetics*, 2002; 30, 102–05.

41. Altmüller J, Palmer LJ, Fischer G, *et al.,* Genomewide scans of complex human diseases: true linkage is hard to find. *American Journal of Human Genetics*, 2001; 69, 936–50.

42. Broeckel U, Hengstenberg C, Mayer B, *et al.,* A comprehensive linkage analysis for myocardial infarction and its related risk factors. *Nature Genetics*, 2002; 30, 210–14.

43. Caulfield M, Munroe P, Pembroke J, *et al.,* Genome-wide mapping of human loci for essential hypertension. *Lancet*, 2003; 361, 2118–23.

44. Williams NM, Norton N, Williams H, *et al.,* A systematic genomewide linkage study in 353 sib pairs with schizophrenia. *American Journal of Human Genetics*, 2003; 73, 1355–67.

45. Xu J, Meyers DA, Ober C, *et al.,* Genomewide screen and identification of gene–gene interactions for asthma-susceptibility loci in three US populations: collaborative study on the genetics of asthma. *American Journal of Human Genetics,* 2001; 68, 1437–46.

46. Wiltshire S, Cardon LR, McCarthy MI, Evaluating the results of genomewide linkage scans of complex traits by locus counting. *American Journal of Human Genetics,* 2002; 71, 1175–82.

47. Kaback MM, Rimoin DL, O'Brien JS, *Tay-Sachs Disease: Screening and Prevention.* New York: Alan R Liss, 1977.

48. Bray F, Sankila R, Ferlay J, *et al.,* Estimates of cancer incidence and mortality in Europe in 1995. *European Journal of Cancer,* 2002; 38, 99–166.

49. Cavalli-Sforza LL, Menozzi P, Piazza A, *The history and geography of human genes.* Princeton, New Jersey: Princeton University Press, 1996.

50. Risch N, Searching for genetic determinants in the new millennium. *Nature,* 200; 405, 847–56.

51. Douglas JA, Boehnke M, Lange K, A multipoint method for detecting genotyping errors and mutations in sibling-pair linkage data. *American Journal of Human Genetics,* 2000; 66, 1287–97.

52. Kennedy JL, Farrer LA, Andreasen NC, *et al.,* The genetics of adult-onset neuropsychiatric disease: complexities and conundra? *Science,* 2003; 302, 822–26.

53. Duggirala R, Williams JT, Williams-Blangero S, *et al.,* A variance component approach to dichotomous trait linkage analysis using a threshold model. *Genetic Epidemiology,* 1997; 14, 987–92.

54. Palmer LJ, Cardon LR, Shaking the tree: mapping complex disease genes with linkage disequilibrium. *Lancet,* 2005; 366, 9492, 1223–34.

55. Wise LH, Lanchbury JS, Lewis CM, Meta-analysis of genome searches. *Annals of Human Genetics,* 1999; 63, 263–72.

56. Levinson DF, Levinson MD, Segurado R, *et al.,* Genome scan meta-analysis of schizophrenia and bipolar disorder, part I: methods and power analysis. *American Journal of Human Genetics,* 2003; 73, 17–33.

57. Roberts SB, MacLean CJ, Neale MC, *et al.,* Replication of linkage studies of complex traits: an examination of variation in location estimates. *American Journal of Human Genetics,* 1999; 65, 876–84.

58. Parrella P, Fazio VM, Gallo AP, *et al.,* Fine mapping of chromosome 3 in uveal melanoma: identification of a minimal region of deletion on chromosomal arm 3p25.1-p25.2. *Cancer Research,* 2003; 63, 8507–10.

59. Nsengimana J, Samani NJ, Hall AS, *et al.,* Enhanced linkage of a locus on chromosome 2 to premature coronary artery disease in the absence of hypercholesterolemia. *European Journal of Human Genetics,* 2007; 15, 3, 313-9.

60. Rankinen T, Zuberi A, Chagnon YC, *et al.,* The human obesity gene map: The 2005 update. *Obesity* (Silver Spring) 2006; 14, 4, 529-644.

61. Ichihara S, Yamada Y, Genetic factors for human obesity. *Cellular and Molecular Life Sciences*, 2008; 65, 7-8, 1086-98.

62 George RA, Smith TD, Callaghan S, *et al.*, General mutation data-bases: analysis and review. *Journal of Medical Genetics*, 2008; 45, 2, 65-70.

63. Rice JP, Saccone NL, Corbett J, Model-based methods for linkage analysis. *Advances in Genetics*, 2008; 60, 155-73.

64. Friedenson B, Breast-cancer genomics. *New England Journal of Medicine*, 2003; 349, 9, 910-1, author reply -1.

65. Calkins ME, Dobie DJ, Cadenhead KS, *et al.*, The consortium on the genetics of endophenotypes in schizophrenia: model recruitment, assessment, and endophenotyping methods for a multisite collaboration. *Schizophrenia Bulletin*, 2007; 33, 1, 33-48.

66. Zheng SL, Sun J, Wiklund F, *et al.*, Cumulative association of five genetic variants with prostate cancer. *New England Journal of Medicine*, 2008; 358, 9, 910-19.

67. Clark AG, Finding genes underlying risk of complex disease by linkage disequilibrium mapping. *Current Option in Genetics and Development*, 2003; 13, 3, 296-302.

THREE

Genetic association studies

Heather J. Cordell, David G. Clayton

Summary

In this chapter, the rationale behind methods of design and analysis of genetic association studies will be reviewed and discussed, and the similarities between genetic association studies and classic epidemiological studies of environmental risk factors will be described. Issues that are specific to studies of genetic risk factors such as the use of certain family-based designs, accounting for different underlying genetic mechanisms and the impact of population history, will also be discussed.

Introduction

Genetic association studies aim to detect association between one or more genetic polymorphisms and a trait, which may be some quantitative characteristic or a discrete attribute or disease. Association differs from linkage in that the same allele, or alleles, are associated with the trait in a similar manner across the whole population, whereas linkage allows different alleles to be associated with the trait in different families. However, genetic associations arise only because modern human populations share common ancestry and it has been argued that association studies are really just a special form of linkage study in which the extended family is the wider population. It is well known that, in linkage analysis, data from distantly related individuals are more powerful for detecting small effects than data from closely related individuals, but this advantage is offset by the fact that, owing to increased possibility for linkage to be destroyed by recombination, linkage extends over shorter distances in distantly related subjects, necessitating a greater density of markers. Association in apparently unrelated subjects represents the extreme of this effect: association analysis has greater power than linkage studies to detect small effects, but requires many more markers to be examined. The fact that association operates only over short distances in the genome has, for a long time, guaranteed association studies an important place in the fine mapping of genetic loci initially detected by linkage. More recently, it has been realised that genetic susceptibility to common complex disorders is likely to involve many genes, most of which have small effects. This fact, together with the identification of large numbers of single nucleotide polymorphisms (SNPs) throughout the genome and rapidly falling genotyping costs, has led to the current importance of association studies in genetic epidemiology. The current principal discovery strategy for complex disease susceptibility genes involves screening large numbers of SNPs for association across the whole genome (Hunter *et al.* 2007; O'Donnell *et al.* 2007; Scuteri *et al.* 2007; Zeggini *et al.* 2007; Wellcome Trust Case Control Consortium 2007).

Although family-based studies still have a place in the study of population association (in addition to linkage), such research has much more in common with classic epidemiological studies of environmental and behavioural risk factors than do linkage studies. Consequently, issues of study design and analysis have more in common with the rest of epidemiology. Parallels with classic epidemiology are also clear if the reasons why association between a genetic polymorphism and a trait could exist in a given population are considered:

- the polymorphism has a causal role;
- the polymorphism has no causal role but is associated with a nearby causal variant;
- the association is due to some underlying stratification or admixture of the population.

In a mixed population, strata may have different environmental exposures, or the founder populations may carry different genetic risks. In these circumstances, any locus whose allele frequencies differ between strata or founder populations will be associated with disease to some extent, regardless of whether or not it is near to a causal locus.

Direct association

The first of these forms of association is termed **direct association**, and studies of direct association target polymorphisms that are themselves putative causal variants. This type of study is the easiest to analyse and the most powerful, but the difficulty is the identification of candidate polymorphisms. It is clear that a mutation in a codon (see Glossary) that leads to an amino acid change is a candidate causal variant. However, it is likely that many causal variants responsible for heritability of common complex disorders will be non-coding. For example, such variants may cause variation in gene regulation and expression or in differential splicing. With the current state of knowledge, not enough is known to predict which variants may have such effects. Thus, direct association studies have the potential to discover only some of the genetic causes of disease and disease-related traits. However, some 10,000-15,000 non-synonymous coding (amino acid changing) SNPs with minor allele frequency exceeding 1% in Europeans have been identified. Screening of a panel of all known common coding variants across the genome was trialled in the Welcome Trust Case-Control Consortium (Burton *et al.* 2007).

Indirect association

In the second type of association, the polymorphism is a surrogate measure of the causal locus and points us towards the real cause. This type of association allows us to search for causal genes in **indirect association** studies. However, indirect associations are even weaker than the direct associations they reflect, and it will usually be necessary to type several surrounding markers in order to have a high chance of picking up the indirect association. These facts render indirect association studies more difficult to analyse, and there is still debate as to the best methods. Indirect studies are also less powerful than direct studies. Finally, in contrast to direct studies, until it can be ascertained that the polymorphisms in a region have been adequately charted, there cannot be a definitive negative result because the possibility that a causal variant exists within the region but is not picked up by the markers chosen cannot be excluded. The latest phase of the human genome project – the International HapMap Project (The International HapMap Consortium, 2003) – had the aim of improving our knowledge in this respect. The completion of the second phase of this study (The International HapMap Consortium, 2005; Frazer *et al.* 2007; Zhang *et al.* 2008), plus rapid recent advances in high-throughput genotyping technology, has enabled 'coverage' of around 80% of the human genome for disease associations in non-African populations using predefined, commercially available marker panels of hundreds of thousands of SNPs designed for genome-wide association studies (Barrett and Cardon, 2006; de Bakker *et al.* 2006; Bexer *et al.* 2007; Zondervan and Cardon, 2007). Historically, most indirect association studies have concentrated on candidate genes, identified either on the basis of their known function or from animal models. Even as whole-genome studies have increasingly been used, candidate gene studies will continue to play an important role. In such studies the SNP discovery and HapMap projects have also made it possible to type markers more densely, not only to improve the chances of detecting true causal associations, but also to increase confidence that negative findings represent true negatives.

Confounded association

The final type of association is due to confounding by stratification and admixture (substructure) within the population. **Confounding** (see Glossary), as in the rest of epidemiology, raises the possibility both of generating false findings (positive confounding) or obscuring true causal associations (negative confounding). However, the problem of unobserved confounding is intractable in classic epidemiology, which dictates limits on the size of causal effect that can be safely inferred from observational studies (Taubes, 1996). Genetic epidemiology offers possibilities for circumventing the difficulty.

The most obvious way of avoiding this difficulty is to carry out association in well mixed, outbred populations. Failing this, any stratification and admixture effects could be reduced by matching (in the design and/or the analysis) on geographical region and on any markers of ethnic origin. In this manner, comparisons can be made, as far as possible, within homogeneous subpopulations. It has been argued that such devices will be sufficient to avoid the rather small confounding effects that might be expected to arise as a result of stratification and admixture (Wacholder *et al.* 2002). However, more recently this view has been questioned. Meta-analyses (Ioannidis *et al.* 2003; Trikalinos *et al.* 2008) have indicated that causal variants for complex disease may, when looked at one at a time, have rather small effects and large studies will be necessary in order to detect them (Dahlman *et al.* 2002; Zeggini *et al.* 2008). Against this background, even modest confounding by stratification and admixture could have important repercussions (Patsopoulos *et al.* 2008). It is not yet known how serious this problem will turn out to be for association studies carried out in Europe or in US Caucasians (Ioannidis *et al.* 2007; Patsopoulos *et al.* 2008) but it has been shown to pose a serious problem in admixed populations such as African-Americans or African-Caribbeans (Hoggart *et al.* 2003; Marchini *et al.* 2004). It should be noted however, that admixture also presents opportunities for gene mapping by exploiting a back-crossing experiment of nature, but such admixture mapping studies are beyond the scope of this chapter (Shriver *et al.* 2003; Ioannidis *et al.* 2007; Seldin, 2007; Zhu *et al.* 2008).

The first method for dealing with confounding by population structure is matching by family; if comparisons are made between siblings with the same parents, confounding by population structure is excluded Spielman and Ewans, 1996). However, such studies are not always very powerful and they are difficult, or even impossible, to carry out on a sufficiently large scale to detect genetic associations reliably (Cardon and Palmer, 2003). The role of such studies in the future will probably be to confirm findings generated by less expensive methods and to answer more complex secondary questions.

The second method for dealing with the problem is to seek genetic markers for population substructure, or **ancestry-informative markers** – loci whose allele frequencies differ between the founder populations (Halder *et al.* 2008). A statistical analysis can then emulate an analysis in which association is measured within strata defined by degree of admixture – the proportion of subjects' genotypes stemming from each founder population (Pritchard and Rosenberg, 1999; Pritchard *et al.* 2000; Satten *et al.* 2001; Hoggart *et al.* 2003; Tsai *et al.* 2005; Price *et al.* 2006; Tang *et al.* 2006). Inevitably, there will be some loss of statistical power as a result of the imperfect measurement of admixture proportions (Divers *et al.* 2007) . This loss of power may be modest for populations in which founder populations are very different and there are good markers of substructure, as in African-Americans (Tian *et al.* 2006), but it remains unclear whether this method can be consistently applied efficiently to control for the smaller differences which might exist, for example, within European populations (Khoury *et al.* 2007; Halder *et al.* 2008).

The third approach to the problem of population substructure is **genomic control** (Devlin and Roeder, 1999; Bacanu *et al.* 2000, 2002; Marchini *et al.* 2004; Price *et al.* 2006; Zheng *et al.* 2006). Confounding is regarded as a random process, potentially affecting all loci, such that the effect of positive confounding is to increase the type 1 error (false positive) rate for association tests. Although conventional tests for association are correct if regarded as tests for association within the population studied, they will have an inflated false positive rate when judged as tests of causal effects in the presence of stratification and/or admixture. Another perspective (more intuitive to geneticists) is that, although subjects in a population-based association study may be regarded as having been independently sampled from the particular population studied, they are not independently sampled when regarded as a sample of all humankind; they are cryptically related because they have been drawn from the same population. As a result, when regarded as tests of the causal null hypothesis, conventional χ^2 tests for association have greater variance than they should have and use of conventional significance levels will lead to a higher false positive rate.

Genomic control is less ambitious than other methods that control for confounding by substructure because it seeks only to control the false positive rate by increasing the threshold required for statistical significance. The factor by which the variance is inflated by confounding can be estimated by typing a large number of unselected markers across the genome and estimating the variance of association test statistics empirically (Marchini et al. 2004). This method is simple to implement. However, no attempt is made to deal with *negative* confounding, which increases the false negative rate, that is, reduces the statistical power of the study. Use of more stringent test criteria to control the false positive rate will accentuate the loss of power. It also remains to be empirically tested whether the distribution of test statistics is inflated by the same multiple regardless of allele frequency and throughout the entire distribution.

It remains to be seen whether the strategy of correcting for confounding by substructure by statistical modelling will be more powerful than accepting some degree of confounding and controlling the resultant type 1 error rate. Much will depend on how serious the problem turns out to be and whether sufficiently informative markers will be identified for the former approach to work efficiently. However, the approaches could turn out to be complementary, with gross effects being addressed by statistical models and surrogate measures of substructure, and more subtle effects, such as those due to cryptic relatedness between cases and/or controls, left to genomic control.

Direct association: patterns of genotype-phenotype relationship

Consider a locus with two alleles (diallelic), directly related either to a quantitative trait, or to a discrete trait such as presence (prevalence) or occurrence (incidence) of a disease. Multi-allelic loci could also be considered, but these lead to more complicated scenarios and generate tests with many degrees of freedom. Even in the simplest diallelic case, different patterns for the genotype-phenotype relationship must be considered. Given that there are three possible genotypes, which have a natural order – 1,1, 1,2 and 2,2 – the question of linearity of the relationship must be considered.

In classic Mendelian genetics of fully penetrant discrete traits, the description of an allele as dominant implies that the corresponding phenotype will occur regardless of the number of copies of the allele carried. In contrast, a recessive allele requires both copies to be present for the corresponding phenotype to be displayed. In a diallelic system, if neither allele is dominant, 1,2 heterozygotes will display some sort of intermediate phenotype. Fisher (1918) used the term 'dominance' in a different way to describe the related concept of linearity of the genotype–phenotype relationship for quantitative traits. In particular, he defined absence of dominance to imply the linear relationship:

$$\text{Mean trait value} = \alpha + \beta x$$

where x codes genotypes 1,1, 1,2, and 2,2 as 0, 1 and 2, respectively. The quantity β represents the additive effect of each copy of allele 2. Because this model predicts that the trait mean for heterozygotes will lie precisely midway between the means for the two types of homozygote, it is easy to see why Fisher identified linearity with absence of dominance, but this idea is based on a stronger model than the earlier concept.

The importance of a simplifying model such as the linear dose–response model above is that the strength of genotype–phenotype relationship is expressed in a single parameter (β) and statistical tests for existence of such a relationship have only one degree of freedom. To extend the model to allow a quite general pattern of relationship an additional parameter to measure deviation from linearity must be introduced. For example a variable z, coded as 0 for homozygotes and 1 for heterozygotes, might be introduced, and consider the model:

$$\text{Mean trait value} = \alpha + \beta x + \gamma z$$

The parameter γ is then said to represent a dominance effect. In this extended model, all patterns of relationship between phenotype mean and the three genotypes are possible, but two parameters now code the association and statistical tests have two degrees of freedom. Consideration of this broader class of models inevitably carries the penalty of reduced power if the pattern of relationship truly is linear. Some have argued that in most cases it would be ideal to constrain the two-parameter model so that the trait mean for heterozygotes cannot lie outside the range delimited by the means for homozygotes. This leads to tests that are intermediate between conventional tests with one and two degrees of freedom (Chiano and Clayton, 1998). In any situation, the choice of the most powerful test depends on the pattern of association that actually exists and, unless confirmatory studies are simply being carried out, this is unknown a priori – a ubiquitous problem for statistical analysis. Perhaps for most complex disease genetics, the model in which heterozygote risk is constrained to lie within the range defined by the two homozygote risks is the best compromise between generality and parsimony. However, such a model is little used, perhaps because of a lack of software implementations.

In order to model gene effects on binary qualitative traits that are not fully penetrant, Wright (1920) introduced the notion of an underlying, unobserved and normally distributed quantitative trait ('liability') governed by Fisher's linear model. The discrete trait is assumed to become manifest when liability exceeds some threshold value. The predictions from Wright's model are very close to those from the logistic regression model, which is the mainstay of statistical analysis in the rest of epidemiology (Breslow and Day, 1980; Clayton and Hills, 1993). With this approach, absence of dominance means that the log odds of response for 1,2 heterozygotes is midway between that for 1,1 and 2,2 homozygotes, and so each allele contributes multiplicatively to the odds. For uncommon traits (as most diseases are), this is nearly the same as the model of multiplicative effects of each allele on *risk*. The multiplicative risk model could be argued to be the natural model for lack of dominance in this context. It has one particularly useful property. **Hardy–Weinberg equilibrium (HWE)** is defined by genotype frequencies consistent with the two alleles being independently sampled from a population of alleles. Genotypes of controls, in a case–control study, should therefore be in HWE. But if disease risk is related to genotype multiplicatively, so that genotype risk may be decomposed into a product of effects of the two alleles, then genotypes of the cases of disease are also expected to be in HWE, with alleles being independently drawn from a population in which the frequency of high-risk alleles is increased. This justifies the widely used practice of counting alleles rather than genotypes in statistical analyses (Sasieni, 1997).

Epistasis

The general issue of dominance relates to the extent to which the joint effect of two alleles carried at a single autosomal locus may be different from the sum (or product in a multiplicative model) of the effects that would be anticipated for each allele independently. A related issue is the degree to which the combined effect of alleles at two or more loci can reasonably be modelled by the individual locus contributions. The fact that inheritance of some traits could only be explained by joint action of two unlinked loci was first demonstrated by Bateson (1909), who termed the phenomenon **epistasis**. In these first examples, variation of phenotype with genotype at one locus was observed only in subjects with certain genotypes at the second locus; other subjects would show no effect. Thus epistasis was defined as the phenomenon of one locus 'masking' the effect of another. Fisher (1918) used a similar term, 'epistacy', to refer to a statistical interaction meaning deviation from additive effects of the two loci on the trait mean. The term 'epistacy' soon evolved into 'epistasis' (Phillips, 1998) with the result that in modern genetics the two uses of the word coexist, often causing confusion (Cordell *et al.* 2001; Cordell, 2002).

Epistasis, defined in Fisher's sense, is scale dependent and, in general, does not have a clear interpretation in terms of mechanism. The interpretation of the causal implications of statistical interaction in epidemiology has been vigorously debated over at least three decades (Siemiatycki and Thomas, 1981; Thompson, 1991). A similar debate continues in relation to interaction between genes and environmental risk factors (Hunter, 2005). Some have argued that the interaction of genes and environment will become a major influence on the epidemiological study of aetiology and on public heath interventions (Khoury and Wagener, 1995; Shpilberg *et al.* 1997; Khoury, 1998; Hunter, 2005), whereas others have been more sceptical (Clayton and McKeigue, 2001). Methods research in this area is ongoing (Dempfle *et al.* 2008).

If interpretation of statistical interaction between genes is problematic there is, nevertheless, an important reason to consider it, which concerns the ability to discover the genes related to complex diseases in the first place. It is argued that, if such genes act together, epistatically, with several genes acting in the same pathway, the marginal effect of each gene when looked at on its own may be small, but might reflect much larger effects of collections of genes (Hoh and Ott, 2003; Moore, 2003; Sieberts and Schadt, 2007). Some authors have even postulated scenarios in which marginal effects are absent altogether (Culverhouse *et al.* 2001). But the latter hypothesis requires one gene to reverse the direction of effect of another – an eventuality that, although possible, is perhaps unlikely to occur widely. Such arguments have led these same researchers to suggest that the analysis of association studies should move away from analysis of genes one at time, focusing instead on pairs or even larger constellations of genes (Sieberts and Schadt, 2007). It is not yet clear whether the gains in effect size realised in practice by considering several genes at a time will be sufficiently pronounced to compensate for the requirement for more stringent correction for the number of hypotheses to be tested (Marchini *et al.* 2005). A further debate concerns the relative merits of recursive partitioning methods that derive from the 'automatic interaction detection' methods of Sonquist and Morgan (1964), originating in the social sciences but now widely used in the computer science and bioinformatics communities, over more standard regression–based approaches.

Indirect association: patterns of linkage disequilibrium

The mapping of susceptibility genes for common complex disorders and genes for other common traits by the indirect method depends on the existence of association, at the population level, between the causal variants and nearby markers. Such association, which is due to proximity of loci on the genome, is termed linkage disequilibrium (LD). Sometimes this term is used to describe any population-wide association between loci, whether due to proximity or to other reason such as population stratification and admixture; however, the term 'allelic association' tends to be used for this more general phenomenon. The term 'gametic phase disequilibrium' is also used to describe allelic association due to proximity. Success of the indirect mapping strategy depends on some understanding of patterns of LD and the forces that determine them – mutation, recombination and population history.

Figure 3.1 shows the genealogy of the same small segment of eight copies of the same chromosome. It is assumed that, if tracked back far enough, they will be descended from a common ancestor, and that the segment is so small that there will have been no recombination within the segment. This latter assumption is necessary because the occurrence of recombination in the sample history complicates things considerably; an adjacent segment separated by a recombination will have an entirely different genealogy above this point. The crosses labelled A, B and C in Figure 3.1 indicate mutations, each one of which will generate a new (diallelic) polymorphism. Assuming that a mutation will not occur in the same locus twice, a mutant allele cannot revert back to wild type, and every copy of the mutant allele in the present population is descended from the same ancestral mutation. The scale for the height of the genealogy is meioses, or generations. In this example, there are four three-locus haplotypes. Labelling the initial allele at each locus as '1' and the new allele created by mutation as '2' (a haplotype is represented as 'locus A allele–locus B allele–locus C allele') these are 1–1–1 (subjects 6, 7 and 8), 1–2–2 (subjects 4 and 5), 2–1–1 (subjects 1 and 2) and 1–2–1 (subject 3). This diagram brings out two key facts:

- alleles that are common in the present sample will represent older mutations;
- the number of different haplotypes increases in direct proportion to the number of polymorphisms, unless some polymorphisms correspond to mutations on the same branch of the genealogy.

Less obvious is the fact that, even under these simplifying assumptions, the pattern and strength of association between polymorphisms is very variable.

The situation presented in the figure represents complete LD between the three loci. This fact is apparent when looking at the loci two at a time; each pair of loci define only three haplotypes. Table 3.1 shows the two-locus haplotype frequencies as 2 x 2 contingency tables. Complete LD between pairs of loci is shown by the fact that at least one cell of the corresponding table is zero, because this is the maximum degree of association possible given the row and column totals. LD decays for three reasons:

1. recombination(s) in the genealogy occurring at some point between the two loci;
2. recurrence of the same mutation;
3. gene conversion (transfer of information between alleles or loci) (Jeffreys and May, 2004).

The first of these is the most important reason for the decay of LD. Because the probability of recombination increases with the distance between the loci, the strength of LD is expected to decline with distance.

Various different measures of pairwise LD have been proposed (Devlin and Risch, 1995), including Lewontin's D' (Lewontin, 1964), which has also been termed the 'association probability' (Morton *et al.* 2001). Lewontin's D' is an important measure for identifying regions in which there has been little recombination and, therefore, in which there is the potential to map causal loci by indirect association studies. However, this measure does not directly determine the power of indirect

Figure 3.1: Genealogy of a sample of eight chromosomes, showing ancestry of three SNPs

See text for details.

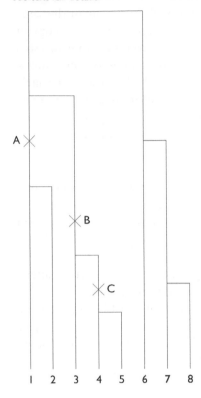

association studies. Formally, the power of tests for indirect association depends largely on the index r^2, the square of the conventional correlation coefficient between the allele at the typed locus, scored 1 or 2, and the allele at the causal locus, scored similarly. The dependence of power on r^2, rather than on any other measure of association, is complete for quantitative traits in the absence of a dominance variance component due to the causal locus (Sham *et al.* 2000). In Table 3.1, the value of r^2 between C and B is 0.56, while that between A and B is only 0.2. The nature of the relationship between r^2 and the power to detect association is such that, if B is causal, it would require a sample size $0.56/0.2 = 2.8$ times as large to detect the indirect association with *A* than to detect the association with C. Table 3.1 clearly demonstrates that, even when loci are in complete disequilibrium (D' = 1.0 in all three sub-tables), the pairwise r^2 values can vary widely, being related to the allele frequencies and to the position of the corresponding mutations in the genealogy.

The phenomenon of LD is also relevant to the ongoing discussion of 'haplotype blocks' (Daly *et al.* 2001; Wall and Pritchard, 2003; Schulze *et al.* 2004). It was suggested that genetic loci across large areas of the genome divide into blocks characterised by little disequilibrium between blocks and limited haplotype diversity within blocks. These two aspects of blocks, physical extent and haplotype diversity, are, in a sense, reflected by the measures D' and r^2, respectively. However, it is important to stress that the two aspects are not necessarily linked, as they are determined by the different random processes of recombination and mutation; both the extent and haplotype diversity of blocks are extremely variable. Furthermore, haplotypic diversity almost inevitably increases as more polymorphisms are discovered.

There has been some discussion as to whether blocks have clear boundaries, coincident with recombination 'hot spots', or whether they arise as a result of purely random forces (Ardlie *et al.* 2002; Wall and Pritchard, 2003, Schulze *et al.* 2004). Sperm typing experiments demonstrate clearly the existence of hot spots (Jeffreys *et al.* 2001) but, undoubtedly, random forces also play an important role. This debate is important in relation to the stability of block structures across populations. It is also relevant to the sharpness of block boundaries. If the extent of haplotypes is determined by random recombination, then all haplotypes

Table 3.1: Pairwise linkage disequilibrium for the eight-chromosome genealogy shown in Figure 3.1

		Locus B			
		1	2	Total	r^2
Locus A	1	3	3	6	
	2	2	0	2	
	Total	5	3		
					0.2

		Locus B			
		1	2	Total	
Locus C	1	5	1	6	
	2	0	2	2	
	Total	5	3		
					0.56

		Locus A			
		1	2	Total	
Locus C	1	4	2	6	
	2	2	0	2	
	Total	6	2		
					0.11

Lewontin's D' measure is 1.0 in all cases.

encompassing a given point in the genome will not be the same length and it would not be surprising to see a few high values of D' extending well outside the main LD block.

The idea of haplotype blocks tends to be linked with the idea of 'haplotype tagging SNPs' (tag SNPs, also called htSNPs) (Johnson *et al.* 2001), largely because these ideas appeared in the literature simultaneously. However, the idea of tag SNPs arose from studies of candidate genes after noting that, after discovering large numbers of SNPs by a combination of database search and exon resequencing, there is usually considerable redundancy – a few tag SNPs capture, in some sense, most of the polymorphism of the gene. Many different methods have been proposed for the choice of tag SNPs (Johnson *et al.* 2001; Stram *et al.* 2003; Chapman *et al.* 2003; Byng *et al.* 2003; Carlson *et al.* 2004). Consideration of the power to detect indirect association via tag SNPs suggest that the important criterion is the coefficient of determination, a generalisation of r^2 to multiple regression models and usually denoted by $\boldsymbol{R^2}$. This quantity measures the ability of a *set* of tag SNPs to predict another dimorphism (Chapman *et al.* 2003; Clayton *et al.* 2004). The R^2 values with which tag SNPs predict the remaining known polymorphisms provide an estimate of the likely ability to predict a causal variant, but, with the limited knowledge of human polymorphism, its accuracy cannot be guaranteed.

Study designs

As already mentioned, familiar epidemiological designs such as population-based case-control or cohort designs (Breslow and Day, 1980; 1987) are often used for genetic association studies. The studies are carried out and the data analysed in a very similar manner too — risk factors such as smoking and obesity are replaced by the presence or absence of a particular genetic polymorphism. Risk may be considered in terms of either a predisposing allele or a predisposing genotype, or in terms of multiple categories of disease risk, such as the risks associated with different alleles at a multi-allelic genetic locus or the risks associated with the three possible genotypes 1,1, 1,2 and 2,2 at a single diallelic locus.

In addition to standard epidemiological designs, several designs have been specifically proposed for genetic studies. Family-based designs such as the case-parent triad design (Falk and Rubinstein, 1987; Schaid and Sommer, 1993), case-parent-grandparent design (Weinberg, 2003) or analysis of general pedigrees have been proposed to counteract the problems of confounding due to population stratification that can occur in case-control (or other population-based) designs (Cardon and Palmer, 2003). In family designs, alleles or genotypes transmitted to affected individuals are compared with untransmitted alleles or genotypes, providing a control sample that is inherently matched to the case sample with regard to population structure. An alternative approach is to use population-based studies, correcting for population stratification by one of the methods described previously (Devlin and Roeder, 1999; Pritchard *et al.* 2000; Satten *et al.* 2001; Price *et al.* 2006). These methods require typing of either a large number of unselected markers or a panel of markers chosen to be highly informative for the type of admixture present in the study population. However, such corrections have become very feasible with the decreasing costs of genotyping and density of available SNP markers (Halder *et al.* 2008). The case-parent triad design typically requires the same number of triads (consisting of a case and two parents) to be typed as the number of cases required in a case-control design (assuming an equal number of controls) to give the same power. Thus a sample of 500 case-parent triads will have approximately the same power as 500 cases and 500 controls, but the case-parent triad design requires 1.5 times the amount of genotyping and may also be more difficult or expensive to collect in the first place (except when family samples have already been collected as part of previous linkage studies). For this reason, the case-control approach is often preferred. However, family-based approaches provide a useful complementary strategy because of their robustness to population stratification and because of their ability to estimate effects such as those due to direct maternal genotype or maternal-fetal interaction (as might arise from influences in utero) and parent-of-origin (imprinting) effects (Weinberg *et al.* 1998; Weinberg, 1999; Sinsheimer *et al.* 2003; Cordell *et al.* 2004). Case-parent triad designs allow such effects to be estimated, but this is at the expense of making rather weak assumptions concerning population distributions of parental genotypes, namely exchangeability of maternal and paternal genotypes. These assumptions may be avoided altogether by use of the case–parent–grandparent design (but such families may be difficult to obtain in practice).

Some designs have been proposed specifically to reduce genotyping costs and effort, for instance by genotyping only those individuals at the extremes of the phenotype distribution (those expected to be most informative for detection of effects). DNA pooling studies (Sham *et al.* 2002; Norton *et al.* 2004) reduce the amount of genotyping by typing DNA pooled from a group of individuals (for example, a group of cases compared with a group of controls) as opposed to genotyping each person individually. Another strategy for reducing genotyping costs is to use the haplotype tagging approach (Johnson *et al.* 2001; Ke and Cardon, 2003; Eyheramendy *et al.* 2007) in which genotypes from an initial sample (say 32 individuals) are used to select a limited number of loci to genotype in a larger sample (of cases and controls for example) (see also Chapter Four). This strategy exploits the indirect association approach to gene mapping. Further savings in cost and efficiency can be obtained by use of a staged strategy (Satagopan and Elston, 2003; Lowe *et al.* 2004; Skol *et al.* 2006).

Table 3.2 summarises the various different designs that are commonly used in genetic association studies. In addition, methods and programs have been developed for performing power and sample size calculations for these studies. These provide a useful resource when comparing designs or calculating the expected power prior to conducting a study. A list of these resources is given in Table 3.3.

Statistical analysis

The analysis of genetic association data obviously depends crucially on the study design used. In the simplest case, familiar methods such as logistic regression, χ^2 tests of association and estimation of odds ratios can be performed. At a single marker, the issue arises as to whether to analyse on the basis of allele counts or genotype counts. For example, consider case-control data for a single diallelic genetic locus as shown in Table 3.4. A simple χ^2 test for independence in this table has two degrees of freedom. Two odds ratios can be calculated: *af/be* (for genotype 2,2 versus 1,1) and *cf/de* (for genotype 1,2 versus 1,1). Alternatively, if there is some prior reason to expect dominance or recessiveness in the effect of allele 2, the top two rows or bottom two rows may be grouped together to provide a χ^2 test on one degree of freedom and an odds ratio of $(a+c)f/(b+d)e$ or $a(d+f)/b(c+e)$, respectively. Another approach might be to perform a test of trend, with a dose-response effect in regard to the number of copies of allele 2. A similar test can be performed by uncoupling the alleles within a genotype and constructing a test in terms of 'case' and 'control' chromosomes, as shown in Table 3.5. A χ^2 test of association on one degree of freedom may be performed on the data in Table 3.5. This procedure assumes that chromosomes or alleles can be considered as independent units (Sasieni, 1997), which essentially means assuming Hardy–Weinberg equilibrium (and, for estimation of effects under the alternative hypothesis, assumes multiplicative effects of alleles). All of these tests

Table 3.2: Study designs for genetic association studies

Design	Details	Advantages	Disadvantages	Statistical analysis method
Cross-sectional	Genotype and phenotype (ie determine disease status or quantitative trait value from) a random sample from population.	Inexpensive. Provides estimate of disease prevalence.	Few affected individuals if disease is rare.	Logistic regression, χ^2 tests of association or linear regression.
Cohort	Genotype subsection of population and follow disease incidence for specified time period.	Provides estimate of disease incidence.	Expensive to follow up. Issues of drop-out.	Survival analysis methods.
Case-control	Genotype specified number of affected ('case') and unaffected ('control') individuals. Cases usually obtained from GPs or disease registries, controls obtained from random population sample or convenience sample.	No need for follow-up. Provides estimates of exposure effects.	Requires careful selection of controls. Potential for confounding (such as from population stratification).	Logistic regression, χ^2 tests of association.
Extreme values	Genotype individuals with extreme (high or low) values of a quantitative trait, as determined from an initial cross-sectional or cohort sample.	Genotype only the most informative individuals, saving on genotyping costs.	No estimate of true genetic effect sizes.	Linear regression, non-parametric or permutation approaches.
Case-parent triads	Genotype affected individuals plus their parents (affected individuals determined from initial cross-sectional, cohort or disease-outcome-based sample).	Robust to population stratification. Can estimate maternal and imprinting effects.	Less powerful than case-control design.	Transmission disequilibrium test (TDT), conditional logistic regression or log-linear models.
Case-parent-grandparent septets	Genotype affected individuals plus their parents and grandparents.	Robust to population stratification. Can estimate maternal and imprinting effects.	Grandparents rarely available.	Log-linear models.
General pedigrees	Genotype random sample or disease-outcome-based sample of families from general population. Phenotype for disease trait or quantitative trait.	Higher power with large families. Sample may already exist from linkage studies.	Expensive to genotype. Many missing individuals.	Pedigree disequilibrium test (PDT), family-based association test (FBAT), quantitative TDT (QTDT).
Case-only	Genotype only affected individuals, obtained from initial cross-sectional, cohort or disease-outcome-based sample.	Most powerful design for detection of interaction effects.	Can only estimate interaction effects. Very sensitive to population stratification.	Logistic regression, χ^2 tests of association.
DNA pooling	Applies to variety of above designs, but genotyping carried out on pools of anywhere between 2 and 100 individuals, rather than on an individual basis.	Potentially inexpensive compared with individual genotyping (but technology still under development).	Hard to estimate different experimental sources of variance.	Estimation of components of variance.

Table 3.3: Resources for power and sample size calculations

Program/Method	Reference	URL
Analytical calculation	Breslow and Day (1987), Risch and Merikangas (1996), Camp (1997; 1999)	
QUANTO	Gauderman (2002a; 2002b)	http://hydra.usc.edu/gxe
Genetic Power Calculator	Purcell et al. (2003)	http://pngu.mgh.harvard.edu/~purcell/gpc/
Stata power and sample size programs	Saunders et al. (2002; 2003)	http://cruk.leeds.ac.uk/katie
TDTPOWER	Knapp (1999)	www.uni-bonn.de/~umt70e/soft.htm
TDTASP	McGinnis (2000), McGinnis et al. (2002)	http://biostatistics.mdanderson.org/SoftwareDownload/
TDT-PC	Chen and Deng (2001)	www.biostat.jhsph.edu/~wmchen/pc.html

can be performed in standard statistical software packages using standard routines and appropriate coding of genotype variables.

Table 3.6 gives references (methodology and software) for some of the statistical analysis methods commonly used in genetic association studies. A useful overview of methodology for genetic association testing may also be found in Balding (2006). Although many tests can be performed in standard statistical analysis packages, some (particularly for analysis of family data) require specialist genetics software or 'add-in' routines. A wide variety of different programs have been developed, therefore those listed in Table 3.6 should be considered only a guide. Although some are designed to be simple and self-explanatory, others may require some degree of specialist training or knowledge of the relevant statistical analysis package.

Table 3.4: Counts of genotypes in a case-control study

Genotype	Cases	Controls
2,2	a	b
1,2	c	d
1,1	e	f

Table 3.5: Counts of chromosomes in case-control study

Allele	Chromosomes of: Cases	Controls
2	2a + c	2b + d
1	2e + c	2f + d

The simplest and most powerful statistical analyses arise in the direct association studies in which causal hypotheses, and hence analyses, are specific to single, typed polymorphisms. However, in indirect studies that exploit LD between typed markers and causal variants, analysis of marker loci one at a time may not be optimal – the r^2 between single markers and the causal locus may be much lower than the R^2 for prediction of the causal locus from a *group* of markers. For such studies, it would be preferable to use multi-locus approaches to analysis. However, these methods are still at a relatively early stage of development.

Multi-locus approaches are generally assumed to involve consideration of haplotypes. Analysis at the haplotype level has the potential to reveal an effect marked by an ancestral haplotype but has two main drawbacks:

1. because the number of haplotypes to consider may be large, the potential gain may be offset by an excessive increase in the degrees of freedom in the test; and
2. haplotype phase will often be uncertain.

There are several ways in which the first problem might be approached. The simplest, and most widely used, is to pool rare haplotypes. This will certainly sacrifice some information, and grouping strategies based on genealogical considerations have been proposed (Seltman *et al.* 2001; Morris, 2005). However, for markers in regions in which LD is strong, it is questionable whether the use of any haplotype information is worth the increase in degrees of freedom. This is because in such circumstances, a simple multiple regression equation with one parameter per marker can achieve prediction of untyped loci with R^2 only slightly worse than haplotype-based predictions (Chapman *et al.* 2003; Clayton *et al.* 2004). This suggests testing for indirect associations either by regression of trait on marker loci, without inclusion of the haplotype-defining interaction terms, or by an appropriate variant of Hotelling's T^2 statistic (Hotelling, 1931; Chapman *et al.* 2003; Fan and Knapp, 2003; Clayton *et al.* 2004). These analyses have the additional attraction of not requiring resolution of haplotype phase and can often be carried out using conventional statistical packages.

When LD is less strong, haplotype analyses remain important, particularly for fine mapping, such as in a stepwise logistic regression strategy (Cordell and Clayton, 2002). It has also been pointed out that long haplotypes, spanning several LD blocks, are particularly important for identifying rare variants (Lin *et al.* 2004), although these would have to have large effects in order to be detectable. The resolution of phase can then present a serious practical problem. Various computational algorithms have been developed to address the phase estimation problem, both in unrelated subjects (Fallin and Schork, 2000; Stephens *et al.* 2001) and in families (O'Connell, 2000). Use of these in a two-stage procedure (Cordell, 2006) (whereby haplotype scoring based on a first haplotype analysis stage are used in a second stage test of association) can be satisfactory in population–based studies, particularly if significance is assessed by permutation arguments. For estimation of relative risks, however, it is generally preferable to consider association and haplotype phase assignment simultaneously (Epstein and Satten, 2003). In family studies, too, simple two–stage approaches break down because information about association is given by transmission patterns, and transmission patterns are relevant to haplotype phase resolution. Even for transmission/disequilibrium studies in which both parents of cases are genotyped successfully at all loci, care is necessary because simply restricting analysis to families in which phase can be assigned can cause bias (Dudbridge *et al.* 2000). This can be avoided by

Table 3.6: Statistical analysis methods for genetic association studies

Analysis method	Approach	References	Software	URL
Logistic regression	Model log odds of disease as linear function of underlying genotype variables.	McCullagh and Nelder (1989), Clayton and Hills (1993)	Standard statistical package such as Stata, SAS, S-Plus, R	www.stata.com/, www.sas.com/, www. insightful.com/products/splus/, www.r-project. org/
χ² test of association	Test for independence of disease status and genetic risk factor.	Clayton and Hills (1993)	Standard statistical package such as Stata, SAS, S-Plus, R	As for logistic regression
Linear regression	Model quantitative trait as linear function of underlying genotype variables.	McCullagh and Nelder (1989)	Standard statistical package such as Stata, SAS, S-Plus, R	As for logistic regression
Survival analysis	Model survivor function/hazard as function of underlying genotype variables.	Breslow and Day (1987), Clayton and Hills (1993)	Standard statistical package such as Stata, SAS, S-Plus, R	As for logistic regression
TDT	Test departure of transmission of alleles from heterozygous parents to affected offspring from null 50:50.	Spielman et al. (1993), Knapp (1999), Clayton (1999), Dudbridge et al. (2000)	Various (e.g. Genehunter, RC-TDT, Genassoc, Transmit, Unphased)	www.broad.mit.edu/ftp/distribution/software/ genehunter/, www.uni-bonn.de/~umt70e/soft. htm, www-gene.cimr.cam.ac.uk/clayton/ software/, www.mrc-bsu.cam.ac.uk/personal/ frank/
Conditional logistic regression	Calculate conditional probability of affected offspring genotypes, given parental genotypes.	Schaid and Sommer (1993), Schaid (1996), Cordell and Clayton (2002), Cordell et al. (2004)	Genassoc, Unphased	www-gene.cimr.cam.ac.uk/clayton/software/, www.mrc-bsu.cam.ac.uk/personal/frank/
Log linear models	Model counts of genotype combinations for mother, father and affected offspring.	Weinberg et al. (1998), Weinberg (1999), Sinsheimer et al. (2003)	Standard statistical package such as Stata, SAS, S-Plus, R	As for logistic regression
Haplotype analysis	Testing and estimation of haplotype effects in case/control or family data	Cordell and Clayton (2002), Cordell (2006), Morris (2005;2006)	Unphased WHAP GENEBPMv2 HAPLO.STATS	www.mrc-bsu.cam.ac.uk/personal/frank/, http://pngu.mgh.harvard.edu/~purcell/#whap, http://mayoresearch.mayo.edu/mayo/research/ biostat/schaid.cfm

Analysis method	Approach	References	Software	URL
PDT	Test departure of transmission of alleles to affected pedigree members from null expectation.	Martin et al. (2000) Dudbridge (2003)	PDT Unphased	www.chg.duke.edu/software/pdt.html, www.mrc-bsu.cam.ac.uk/personal/frank/
FBAT	Test for association/linkage between disease phenotypes and haplotypes by using family-based controls.	Laird et al. (2000), Lake et al. (2000), Lunetta et al. (2000), Horvath et al. (2001)	FBAT PBAT P2BAT	www.biostat.harvard.edu/~fbat/fbat.htm, www.biostat.harvard.edu/~clange/default.htm, http://people.fas.harvard.edu/~tjhoffm/pbatR. html
QTDT	Linkage disequilibrium analysis of quantitative and qualitative traits based on variance components.	Abecasis et al. (2000a), Abecasis et al. (2000b)	QTDT	www.sph.umich.edu/csg/abecasis/QTDT/
DNA pooling	Test for differences in allele frequencies in different pooled samples while estimating components of variance due to experimental error.	Darvasi and Soller (1994), Barcellos et al. (1997), Bader et al. (2001), Sham et al. (2002), Barratt et al. (2002)	Standard statistical package such as Stata, SAS, S-Plus, R	As for logistic regression

judicious selection of the information used in the analysis (Cordell and Clayton, 2002), albeit with some loss of information. Alternatively, as in population-based studies, phase uncertainty can be allowed for explicitly in the association analysis (Clayton, 1999). The problem of uncertain phase may be avoided altogether by use of molecular methods for haplotyping (Michalatos-Beloin *et al.* 1996; Eitan and Kashi, 2002) but such methods usually have lower throughput and are more expensive than methods that yield only the diplotype.

In addition to associations between phenotypes and single genes, interaction effects between genes or between genes and environment can also be studied. After taking account of the vast increase in the number of tests that could potentially be carried out, the power to detect interactions is generally expected to be low. However, power can be increased if it is possible to safely assume independence between genes, or between a gene and an environmental exposure, within the population as a whole and, therefore, within controls. Evidence for statistical interaction can then be obtained from examination of cases only (Piegorsch *et al.* 1994; Weinberg and Umbach, 2000). However, as has been stressed, the relationship between statistical and biological interactions (functional interaction between proteins, for example) is complex. Such analyses are more relevant to prediction of disease risk than to the elucidation of the underlying trait pathogenesis (Siemiatycki and Thomas, 1981; Thompson, 1991; Cordell, 2002).

Significance and importance

It has become increasingly clear that the standards of statistical proof that have become acceptable in the general biomedical literature are not appropriate for genetic association studies. It has been recognised that there is something akin to a multiple testing problem that pervades the discipline, although there has been no clear consensus on how it should be dealt with. Classical approaches such as the Bonferroni corrections are not appropriate because it is not the number of tests carried out in any one investigation that is the important consideration. Rather, it is the fact that the vast majority of loci tested will not be associated, so that even a small false positive probability will lead to the situation in which most positive results will turn out to be false. Thus, it is the probability of association that needs to be taken into account, rather than the number of tests (Rice *et al.* 2008). Thus, methods based around the application of Bayes theorem may be more appropriate (Wacholder *et al.* 2004; Thomas and Clayton, 2004). When prior probability of association is known, this allows the calculation of the posterior probability that an association is genuine. However, the equations require knowledge not only of the prior probability of association, but also of the distribution of the size of effects that will be encountered (Rice *et al.* 2008).

In gene expression array studies, so many tests are carried out simultaneously that these unknowns can be estimated within the experiment, so that empirical Bayes methods can be used (Efron and Tibshirani, 2002; Storey and Tibshirani, 2003). As genome-wide association studies with many thousands of SNPs have become feasible, such methods have become appropriate for association studies (Sabatti *et al.* 2003; Dudbridge and Koeleman, 2004; Ziegler *et al.* 2008), but in studies of candidate regions, the prior probabilities that determine appropriate standards of evidence remain largely subjective. However, such considerations show that, given the small a priori probability that any genetic locus is associated with disease, taken together with the small effect sizes that seem to be typical and the inadequate study sizes that have also been typical, it should not be at all surprising that most findings judged positive using conventional levels of statistical significance have not been replicated (Ioannidis *et al.* 2003).

Some would respond to this situation by pointing to the very low population-attributable fractions that correspond to these small genetic effects, and asking whether there is any utility in their discovery. However, no one would claim that the interventions that will follow from advances in genetic epidemiology will simply correct the less beneficial genetic variation. Instead, the important role of such study will be the elucidation of mechanisms. In epidemiology, the role of genetic variation can be important in establishing the causal nature of environmental associations in which intervention could have major effects (Ebrahim and Davey Smith, 2008; see Chapter Seven).

References

Abecasis G, Cardon L, Cookson W, A general test of association for quantitative traits in nuclear families, *American Journal of Human Genetics,* 2000a; 66, 279–92.

Abecasis G, Cookson W, Cardon L, Pedigree tests of transmission disequilibrium. *European Journal of Human Genetics,* 2000b; 8, 545–51.

Ardlie K, Kruglyak L, Seielstad, M, Patterns of linkage disequilibrium in the human genome. *Nature Reviews Genetics,* 2002; 3, 299–309.

Bacanu S, Devlin B, Roeder K, The power of genomic control. *American Journal of Human Genetics,* 2000; 66, 1933–44.

Bacanu S, Devlin B, Roeder K, Association studies for quantitative traits in structured populations. *Genetic Epidemiology,* 2002; 22, 78–93.

Bader J, Bansal A, Sham P, Efficient SNP-based tests of association for quantitative phenotypes using pooled DNA. *GeneScreen,* 2001; 1, 143–50.

Balding D, A tutorial on statistical methods for population association studies. *Nature Reviews Genetics,* 2006; 7, 781–91.

Barcellos L, Klitz W, Field, L, *et al.,* Association mapping of disease loci, by use of a pooled DNA genomic screen. *American Journal of Human Genetics,* 1997; 61, 734–47.

Barrett JC, Cardon LR, Evaluating coverage of genome-wide association studies. *Nature Genetics,* 2006; 38, 659 – 662.

Barratt B, Payne F, Rance H, *et al.,* Identification of the sources of error in allele frequency estimations from pooled DNA indicates an optimal experimental design. *Annals of Human Genetics,* 2002; 66, 393–405.

Bateson, W, *Mendel's principles of heredity.* Cambridge: Cambridge University Press, 1909.

Beyer A, Bandyopadhyay S, Ideker T, Integrating physical and genetic maps: from genomes to interaction networks. *Nature Reviews Genetics,* 2007; 8, 699–710.

Breslow N, Day N, *Statistical Methods in Cancer Research. Volume I – The Analysis of Case–Control Studies.* Lyon: IARC Scientific Publications, 1980.

Breslow N, Day N, *Statistical Methods in Cancer Research. Volume II – The Design and Analysis of Cohort Studies,* Lyon: IARC Scientific Publications, 1987.

Burton PR, Clayton DG, Cardon LR, *et al.,* Association scan of 14,500 nonsynonymous SNPs in four diseases identifies autoimmunity variants. *Nature Genetics,* 2007; 39, 1329-37.

Byng MC, Whittaker JC, Cuthbert AP, *et al.,* SNP subset selection for genetic association studies. *Annals of Human Genetics,* 2003; 67, 543–56.

Camp N, Genomewide transmission/disequilibrium testing – consideration of the genotypic relative risks at disease loci. *American Journal of Human Genetics,* 1997; 61, 1424–30.

Camp N, Genomewide transmission/disequilibrium testing: a correction. *American Journal of Human Genetics,* 1999; 64, 1485–7.

Cardon LR, Palmer L, Population stratification and spurious allelic association. *Lancet,* 2003; 361, 598–604.

Carlson CS, Eberle MA, Rieder MJ, *et al.,* Selecting a maximally informative set of single-nucleotide polymorphisms for association analyses using linkage disequilibrium. *American Journal of Human Genetics,* 2004; 74, 106–20.

Chapman JM, Cooper JD, Todd JA, *et al.,* Detecting disease associations due to linkage disequilibrium using haplotype tags: A class of tests and the determinants of statistical power. *Human Heredity,* 2003; 56, 18–31.

Chen W, Deng H, A general and accurate approach for computing the statistical power of the transmission disequilibrium test for complex disease genes. *Genetic Epidemiology,* 2001; 21, 53–67.

Chiano M, Clayton D, Genotype relative risks under ordered restriction. *Genetic Epidemiology,* 1998; 15, 135–46.

Clayton D, A generalization of the transmission/disequilibrium test for uncertain-haplotype transmission. *American Journal of Human Genetics,* 1999; 65, 1170–7.

Clayton D, Chapman J, Cooper J, The use of unphased multilocus genotype data in indirect association studies. *Genetic Epidemiology,* 2004; 27, 415–28.

Clayton, D, Hills M, *Statistical Models in Epidemiology,* Oxford: Oxford University Press, 1993.

Clayton D, McKeigue P, Epidemiological methods for studying genes and environmental factors in complex diseases. *Lancet,* 2001; 358, 1357–60.

Cordell H, Epistasis: what it means, what it doesn't mean, and statistical methods to detect it in humans. *Human Molecular Genetics,* 2002; 11, 2463–8.

Cordell H, Estimation and testing of genotype and haplotype effects in case-control studies: comparison of weighted regression and multiple imputation procedures. *Genetic Epidemiology*, 2006; 30, 259–75.

Cordell H, Barratt B, Clayton D, Case/pseudo-control analysis in genetic association studies: a unified framework for detection of genotype and haplotype associations, gene-gene and gene-environment interactions and parent-of-origin effects. *Genetic Epidemiology*, 2004; 26, 167–85.

Cordell H, Clayton D, A unified stepwise regression procedure for evaluating the relative effects of polymorphisms within a gene using case/control or family data: application to *HLA* in type 1 diabetes. *American Journal of Human Genetics*, 2002; 70, 124–41.

Cordell H, Todd J, Hill N, *et al.*, Statistical modeling of interlocus interactions in a complex disease: Rejection of the multiplicative model of epistasis in type 1 diabetes. *Genetics*, 2001; 158, 357–67.

Culverhouse R, Suarez B, Lin J, *et al.*, A perspective on epistasis: limits of models displaying no main effects. *American Journal of Human Genetics*, 2001; 70, 461–71.

Dahlman I, Eaves IA, Kosoy R, *et al.*, (2002) Parameters for reliable results in genetic association studies in common disease. *Nature Genetics*, 2002; 30, 149–50.

Daly M, Rioux J, Schaffer S, *et al.*, High-resolution haplotype structure in the human genome. *Nature Genetics*, 2001; 29, 229–32.

Darvasi A, Soller M, Selective DNA pooling for determination of linkage between a molecular markers and a quantitative trait locus. *Genetics*, 1994; 138, 1365–73.

Davey Smith G, Ebrahim S, Mendelian randomisation. *International Journal of Epidemiology*, 2003; 32, 1–22.

De Bakker PI, Graham RR, Altshuler D, et al., Transferability of tag SNPs to capture common genetic variation in DNA repair genes across multiple populations. Pacific Symposium on Biocomputing, 2006; 478-86.

Dempfle A, Scherag A, Hein R, *et al.*, Gene-environment interactions for complex traits: definitions, methodological requirements and challenges. *European Journal of Human Genetics*, 2008; 16, 1164–1172.

Devlin B, Risch N, A comparison of linkage disequilibrium measures for fine–scale mapping. *Genomic*, 1995; 29, 311–22.

Devlin, B, Roeder, K, Genomic control for association studies. *Biometrics,*1999; 55, 997–1004.

Divers J, Vaughan LK, Padilla MA, *et al.*, Correcting for measurement error in individual ancestry estimates in structured association tests. *Genetics*, 2007; 176, 1823–33.

Dudbridge F, Pedigree disequilibrium tests for multilocus haplotypes. *Genetic Epidemiology*, 2003; 25, 115–21.

Dudbridge F, Koeleman BP, Efficient computation of significance levels for multiple associations in large studies of correlated data, including genomewide association studies. *American Journal of Human Genetics*, 2004; 75, 424-35.

Dudbridge F, Koeleman B, Todd J, Clayton D, Unbiased application of the transmission/disequilibrium test to multilocus haplotypes. *American Journal of Human Genetics*, 2000; 66, 2009–12.

Ebrahim S, Davey Smith G, Mendelian randomization: can genetic epidemiology help redress the failures of observational epidemiology? *Human Genetics*, 2008; 123, 15-33.

Efron B, Tibshirani R, Empirical Bayes methods and false discovery rates for microarrays. *Genetic Epidemiology*, 2002; 23, 70–86.

Eitan Y, Kashi Y, Direct micro-haplotyping by multiple double PCR amplifications of specific alleles (md-pasa). *Nucleic Acids Research*, 2002; 30, 12, e62.

Epstein M, Satten G, Inference on haplotype effects in case-control studies using unphased genotype data. *American Journal of Human Genetics*, 2003; 73, 6, 1316–29.

Evans DM, Marchini J, Morris AP, *et al.*, Two-stage two-locus models in genome-wide association. *PLoS Genet*, 2006; 2, e157.

Eyheramendy S, Marchini J, McVean G, *et al.*, A model-based approach to capture genetic variation for future association studies. *Genome Research*, 2007; 17, 88-95.

Falk C, Rubinstein P, Haplotype relative risks: An easy and reliable way to construct a proper control sample for risk calculations. *Annals of Human Genetics*, 1987; 51, 3, 227–33.

Fallin D, Schork N, Accuracy of haplotype frequency estimation for biallelic loci, via the expectation-maximization algorithm for unphased diploid genotype data. *American Journal of Human Genetics*, 2000; 67, 4, 947–59.

Fan R, Knapp M, Genome association studies of complex diseases by case-control designs. *American Journal of Human Genetics*, 2003; 72, 4, 850–68.

Fisher R, The correlation between relatives on the supposition of Mendelian inheritance. *Transactions of the Royal Society of Edinburgh*, 1918; 52, 399–433.

Frazer KA, Ballinger DG, Cox DR, *et al.*, A second generation human haplotype map of over 3.1 million SNPs. *Nature*, 2007; 449, 851-61.

Gauderman W, Sample size calculations for matched case-control studies of gene-environment interaction. *Statistics in Medicine*, 2002a; 21, 1, 35–50.

Gauderman W, Sample size requirements for association studies of gene-gene interaction. *American Journal of Epidemiology*, 2002b; 155, 5, 478–84.

Halder I, Shriver M, Thomas M, *et al.*, A panel of ancestry informative markers for estimating individual biogeographical ancestry and admixture from four continents: utility and applications. *Human Mutation*, 2008; 29, 648-58.

Hoggart C, Parra E, Shriver M, *et al.*, Control of confounding of genetic associations in stratified populations. *American Journal of Human Genetics*, 2003; 72, 6, 1492–504.

Hoh J, Ott J, Mathematical multi-locus approaches to localizing complex human trait genes. *Nature Reviews Genetics*, 2003; 4, 9, 701–9.

Horvath S, Xu X, Laird N, The family based association test method: strategies for studying general genotype-phenotype associations. *European Journal of Human Genetics*, 2001; 9, 4, 301–6.

Hotelling H, The generalization of Student's ratio. *Annals of Mathematical Statistics*, 1931; 2, 3, 360–78.

Hunter DJ, Gene-environment interactions in human diseases. *Nature Reviews Genetics*, 2005; 6, 287-98.

Hunter DJ, Kraft P, Jacobs KB, *et al.*, A genome-wide association study identifies alleles in FGFR2 associated with risk of sporadic postmenopausal breast cancer. *Nature Genetics*, 2007; 39, 870-4.

Ioannidis JP, Patsopoulos NA, Evangelou E, Heterogeneity in meta-analyses of genome-wide association investigations. *PLoS ONE*, 2007; 2, e841.

Ioannidis J, Trikalinos T, Ntzani E, *et al.*, Genetic associations in large versus small studies: an empirical assessment. *Lancet*, 2003; 361, 9357, 567–71.

Jeffreys AJ, Kauppi L, Neumann H, Intensely punctate meiotic recombination in the class II region of the major histocompatibilty complex. *Nature Genetics*, 2001; 29, 2, 217–22.

Jeffreys AJ, May C, Intense and highly localized gene conversion activity in human meiotic crossover hot spots. *Nature Genetics*, 2004; 36, 427, 151–6.

Johnson G, Esposito L, Barratt B, *et al.*, Haplotype tagging for the identification of common disease genes. *Nature Genetics*, 2001; 29, 2, 233–7.

Ke X, Cardon LR, Efficient selective screening of haplotype tag SNPs. *Bioinformatics*, 2003; 19, 287-8.

Khoury M, Genetic and epidemiological approaches to the search for gene-environment interaction: the case of osteoporosis. *American Journal of Epidemiology*, 1998; 147, 1, 1–2.

Khoury MJ, Little J, Gwinn M, et al., On the synthesis and interpretation of consistent but weak gene-disease associations in the era of genome-wide association studies. International Journal Epidemiology, 2007; 36, 439-45.

Khoury M, Wagener D, Epidemiological evaluation of the use of genetics to improve the predictive value of disease risk factors. *American Journal of Human Genetics*, 1995; 56, 4, 835–44.

Knapp M, A note on power approximations for the transmission/disequilibrium test. *American Journal of Human Genetics*, 1999; 64, 4, 861–70.

Laird N, Horvath S, Xu X, Implementing a unified approach to family based tests of association. *Genetic Epidemiology*, 2000; 19, S1, S36–S42.

Lake S, Blacker D, Laird N, Family-based tests of association in the presence of linkage. *American Journal of Human Genetics*, 2000; 67, 6, 1515–25.

Lewontin, R, The interaction of selection and linkage I. General considerations. *Genetics*, 1964; 49, 1, 49–67.

—

Lin S, Chakravarti A, Cutler DJ, Exhaustive allelic transmission disequilibrium tests as a new approach to genome-wide association studies. *Nature Genetics*, 2004: 36, 11, 1181–8.

Lowe, C, Cooper J, Chapman J, *et al.*, Cost-effective analysis of candidate genes using htSNPs: A staged approach. *Genes and Immunity*, 2004; 5, 4, 301–5.

Lunetta K, Faraone S, Biederman J, *et al.*, Family-based tests of association and linkage that use unaffected sibs, covariates, and interactions. *American Journal of Human Genetics*, 2000; 66, 2, 605–14.

Marchini J, Cardon LR, Phillips MS, *et al.*, The effects of human population structure on large genetic association studies. *Nature Genetics*, 2004; 36, 512-7.

Marchini J, Donnelly P, Cardon L, (2005) Genome-wide strategies for detecting multiple loci that influence complex diseases. *Nature Genetics*, 2005; 37, 4, 413–17.

Martin E, Monks S, Warren L, *et al.*, A test for linkage and association in general pedigrees: the pedigree disequilibrium test. *American Journal of Human Genetics*, 2000; 67, 1, 146–54.

McCullagh P, Nelder J, *Generalized Linear Models*. London: Chapman & Hall, 1989.

McGinnis R, General equations for Pt, Ps, and the power of the TDT and the affected-sib-pair test. *American Journal of Human Genetics*, 2000; 67, 5, 1340–7.

McGinnis R, Shifman S, Darvasi A, Power and efficiency of the TDT and case-control design for association scans. *Behavior Genetics*, 2002; 32, 2, 135–44.

Michalatos-Beloin S, Tishkoff S, Bentley K, *et al.*, (1996) Molecular haplotyping of genetic markers 10 kb apart by allele-specific long-range PCR. *Nucleic Acids Research*, 1996; 24, 23, 4841–3.

Moore J, The ubiquitous nature of epistasis in determining susceptibility to common human diseases. *Human Heredity*, 2003; 56, 1-3, 73–82.

Morris A, Direct analysis of unphased snp genotype data in population-based association studies via bayesian partition modelling of haplotypes. *Genetic Epidemiology*, 2005; 29, 2, 91–107.

Morris A, A flexible bayesian framework for modeling haplotype association with disease, allowing for dominance effects of the underlying causative variants. *American Journal of Human Genetics*, 2006; 79, 4, 679–94.

Morton N, Zhang W, Taillon-Miller P, *et al.*, The optimal measure of allelic association. *Proceedings of the National Academy of Sciences of the United States of America*, 2001; 98, 9, 5217–21.

Norton N, Williams NM, O'Donovan MC, *et al.*, DNA pooling as a tool for large-scale association studies in complex traits. *Annals of Medicine*, 2004; 36, 146-52.

O'Connell J, Zero-recombinant haplotyping: application of fine mapping usings SNPs. *Genetic Epidemiology*, 2000; 19, S1, S64–S70.

O'Donnell CJ, Cupples LA, D'Agostino RB, *et al.*, Genome-wide association study for subclinical atherosclerosis in major arterial territories in the NHLBI's Framingham Heart Study. *BMC Medical Genetics*, 2007; 8 Suppl 1, S4.

Patsopoulos NA, Evangelou E, Ioannidis JP, Sensitivity of between-study heterogeneity in meta-analysis: proposed metrics and empirical evaluation. *International Journal of Epidemiology*, 2008; 37, 1148–57.

Phillips P, The language of gene interaction. *Genetics*, 1998; 149, 3, 1167–71.

Piegorsch W, Weinberg C, Taylor J, Non-hierarchical logistic models and case-only designs for assessing susceptibility in population-based case-control studies. *Statistics in Medicine*, 1994; 13, 2, 153–62.

Price A, Patterson N, Plenge R, *et al.*, Principal components analysis corrects for stratification in genome-wide association studies. *Nature Genetics*, 2006; 38, 8, 904–9.

Pritchard J, Rosenberg N, Use of unlinked genetic markers to detect population stratification in association studies. *American Journal of Human Genetics*, 1999; 65, 1, 220–228.

Pritchard J, Stephens M, Rosenberg N, *et al.*, Association mapping in structured populations. *American Journal of Human Genetics*, 2000; 67, 1, 170–81.

Purcell, S, Cherny S, Sham P, Genetic power calculator: design of linkage and association genetic mapping studies of complex traits. *Bioinformatics*, 2003; 19, 1, 149–50.

Rice TK, Schork NJ, Rao DC, Methods for handling multiple testing. *Advances in Genetics*, 2008; 60, 293-308.

Risch N, Merikangas K, The future of genetic studies of complex human diseases. *Science*, 1996; 273, 5281, 1516–17.

Sabatti C, Service S, Freimer N, False discovery rate in linkage and association genome screens for complex disorders. *Genetics*, 2003; 164, 2, 829–33.

Sasieni, P, From genotypes to genes: doubling the sample size. *Biometrics*, 1997; 53, 4, 1253–61.

Satagopan J, Elston, R, Optimal two-stage genotyping in population-based association studies. *Genetic Epidemiology*, 2003; 25, 2, 149–57.

Satten G, Flanders W, Yang Q, Accounting for unmeasured population substructure in case–control studies of genetic association using a novel latent–class model. *American Journal of Human Genetics*, 2001; 68, 2, 466–77.

Saunders C, Bishop D, Barrett J, (2002) Power and sample size calculations for studies of gene-gene and gene-environment interactions. *Genetic Epidemiology*, 2002; 23, 302–3.

Saunders C, Bishop D, Barrett J, Sample size calculations for main effects and interactions in case-control studies using Stata's nchi2 and npnchi2 functions. *The Stata Journal*, 2003; 3, 1, 1–10.

Schaid D, General score tests for associations of genetic markers with disease using cases and their parents. *Genetic Epidemiology*, 1996; 13, 5, 423–49.

Schaid D, Sommer S, Genotype relative risks: methods for design and analysis of candidate-gene association studies. *American Journal of Human Genetics*, 1993; 53, 5, 1114–26.

Schulze TG, Zhang K, Chen YS, *et al.*, Defining haplotype blocks and tag single-nucleotide polymorphisms in the human genome. *Human Molecular Genetics*, 2004; 13, 335-42.

Scuteri A, Sanna S, Chen WM, *et al.*, Genome-wide association scan shows genetic variants in the FTO gene are associated with obesity-related traits. *PLoS Genetics*, 2007; 3, e115.

Seldin MF, Admixture mapping as a tool in gene discovery. *Current Opinion in Genetics and Development*, 2007; 17, 177-81.

Seltman H, Roeder K, Devlin B, Transmission/disequilibrium test meets measured haplotype analysis: family-based association analysis guided by evolution of haplotypes. *American Journal of Human Genetics*, 2001; 68, 5, 1250–63.

Sham P, Bader J, Craig I, *et al.*, DNA pooling: a tool for large-scale association studies. *Nature Reviews Genetics*, 2002; 3, 3, 862–71.

Sham PC, Cherny SS, Purcell S, *et al.*, Power of linkage versus association analysis of quantitative traits, by use of variance-components models, for sibship data. *American Journal of Human Genetics*, 2000; 66, 5, 1616–30.

Shpilberg O, Dorman J, Ferrel M, *et al.*, The next stage: molecular epidemiology. *Journal of Clinical Epidemiology*, 1997; 50, 6, 635–38.

Shriver MD, Parra EJ, Dios S, *et al.*, Skin pigmentation, biogeographical ancestry and admixture mapping. *Human Genetics*, 2003; 112, 387-99.

Sieberts SK, Schadt EE, Moving toward a system genetics view of disease. *Mammalian Genome*, 2007; 18, 389-401.

Siemiatycki J, Thomas D, Biological models and statistical interactions: an example from multistage carcinogenesis. *International Journal of Epidemiology*, 1981; 10, 4, 383–7.

Sinsheimer J, Palmer C, Woodward J, Detecting genotype combinations that increase risk for disease: maternal-fetal genotype incompatibility test. *Genetic Epidemiology*, 2003; 24, 1, 1–13.

Skol A, Scott LJ, Abecasis G, *et al.*, Joint analysis is more efficient than replication-based analysis for two-stage genome-wide association studies. *Nature Genetics*, 2006; 38, 2, 209–13.

Sonquist J, Morgan J, *The detection of interaction effects, volume Monograph 35 of Survey Research Center*. Michigan: Institute of Social Research, University of Michigan, 1964.

Spielman R, McGinnis R, Ewens W, Transmission test for linkage disequilibrium: The insulin gene region and insulin–dependent diabetes mellitus. *American Journal of Human Genetics*, 1993; 52, 3, 506–16.

Spielman R, Ewans W, The TDT and other family-based tests for linkage disequilibrium and association. *American Journal of Human Genetics*, 1996; 59, 983-9.

Stephens M, Smith N, Donnelly P, A new statistical method for haplotype reconstruction from population data. *American Journal of Human Genetics*, 2001; 68, 4, 978–89.

Storey J, Tibshirani R, Statistical significance for genomewide studies. *Proceedings of the National Academy of Sciences of the United States of America*, 2003; 100, 16, 9440–5.

Stram D, Haiman C, Altshuler D, *et al.*, Choosing haplotype tagging SNPs based on unphased genotype data using a preliminary sample of unrelated subjects with an example from the multiethnic cohort study. *Human Heredity*, 2003; 55, 1, 27–36.

Tang H, Coram M, Wang P, *et al.*, Reconstructing genetic ancestry blocks in admixed individuals. *American Journal of Human Genetics*, 2006; 79, 1–12.

Taubes G, Epidemiology faces its limits. *Science*, 1996; 269, 5221, 164–9.

The International HapMap Consortium, The International HapMap project. *Nature*, 2003; 426, 6968, 789–96.

The International HapMap Consortium, A haplotype map of the human genome. *Nature*, 2005; 437, 7063, 1299–1320.

Thomas D, Clayton D, Betting odds and genetic associations. *Journal of the National Cancer Institute*, 2004; 96, 6, 421–3.

Thompson W, Effect modification and the limits of biological inference from epidemiologic data. *Journal of Clinical Epidemiology*, 1991; 44, 3, 221–32.

Tian C, Hinds DA, Shigeta R, *et al.*, A genomewide single-nucleotide-polymorphism panel with high ancestry information for African American admixture mapping. *American Journal of Human Genetics*, 2006; 79, 640-9.

Trikalinos TA, Salanti G, Zintzaras E, *et al.*, Meta-analysis methods. *Advances in Genetics*, 2008; 60, 311-34.

Tsai HJ, Choudhry S, Naqvi M, *et al.*, Comparison of three methods to estimate genetic ancestry and control for stratification in genetic association studies among admixed populations. *Human Genetics*, 2005; 118, 424-33.

Wacholder S, Chanock S, Garcia-Closas M, *et al.*, Assessing the probability of false positive reports in molecular epidemiology studies. *Journal of the National Cancer Institute*, 2004; 96, 6, 434–42.

Wacholder S, Rothman N, Caporaso N, Counterpoint: bias from population stratification is not a major threat to the validity of conclusions from epidemiological studies of common polymorphisms and cancer. *Cancer Epidemiology Biomarkers and Prevention*, 2002; 11, 6, 513–20.

Wall J, Pritchard J, Haplotype blocks and linkage disequilibrium in the human genome. *Nature Reviews Genetics*, 2003; 4, 8, 587–97.

Weinberg C, Methods for detection of parent-of-origin effects in genetic studies of case-parents triads. *American Journal of Human Genetics*, 1999; 65, 1, 229–35.

Weinberg C, Studying parents and grandparents to assess genetic contributions to early-onset disease. *American Journal of Human Genetics*, 2003; 72, 2, 438–47.

Weinberg C, Umbach D, Choosing a retrospective design to assess joint genetic and environmental contributions to risk. *American Journal of Epidemiology*, 2000; 152, 3, 197–203.

Weinberg C, Wilcox A, Lie R, A log-linear approach to case-parent-triad data: assessing effects of disease genes that act either directly or through maternal effects and that may be subject to parental imprinting. *American Journal of Human Genetics*, 1998; 62, 4, 969–78.

Wellcome Trust Case Control Consortium, Genome-wide association study of 14,000 cases of seven common diseases and 3,000 shared controls. *Nature*, 2007; 447, 661-78.

Wright S, The relative importance of heredity and environment in determining the piebald pattern of guinea–pigs. *Proceedings of the National Academy of Sciences of the United States of America*, 1920; 6, 6, 320–2.

Zeggini E, Scott LJ, Saxena R, *et al.*, Meta-analysis of genome-wide association data and large-scale replication identifies additional susceptibility loci for type 2 diabetes. *Nature Genetics*, 2008; 40, 638-45.

Zeggini E, Weedon MN, Lindgren CM, *et al.*, Replication of genome-wide association signals in UK samples reveals risk loci for type 2 diabetes. *Science*, 2007; 316, 1336-41.

Zhang W, Ratain MJ, Dolan ME, The HapMap resource is providing new insights into ourselves and its application to pharmacogenomics. *Bioinformation Biology Insights*, 2008; 2, 15-23.

Zheng G, Freidlin B, Gastwirth JL, Robust genomic control for association studies. *American Journal of Human Genetics*, 2006; 78, 350-6.

Zhu X, Tang H, Risch N, Admixture mapping and the role of population structure for localizing disease genes. *Advances in Genetics*, 2008; 60, 547-69.

Ziegler A, Konig IR, Thompson JR, Biostatistical aspects of genome-wide association studies. *Biometrical Journal*, 2008; 50, 8-28.

Zondervan KT, Cardon LR, Designing candidate gene and genome-wide case-control association studies. *Nature Protocols*, 2007; 2, 2492-501.

FOUR

Mapping complex disease genes using linkage disequilibrium and genome-wide association scans

Lyle J. Palmer, Nicholas J. Timpson, David M. Evans,
George Davey Smith, Lon R. Cardon

Summary

Remarkable advances have occurred recently in our ability to detect genetic polymorphisms contributing to susceptibility to complex human disease. The technology for detecting and scoring single nucleotide polymorphisms (SNPs) has undergone rapid development, yielding extensive catalogues of these polymorphisms across the genome. Population-based maps of the correlations among SNPs (linkage disequilibrium) have been developed to accelerate the discovery of variants contributing to complex diseases in humans, and have been applied in genome-wide association studies. These advances coincide with an increasing recognition of the importance of very large sample sizes for studying genetic effects and have resulted in the discovery of over 150 validated new genes for complex phenotypes since early 2007. This chapter reviews the state of knowledge about the structure of the human genome as related to SNPs and linkage disequilibrium, discusses the application of this knowledge to mapping complex disease genes using genome-wide association studies, considers related methodological and study design issues, and considers the future of genetic association studies.

Introduction

Genetic analysis at the scale of the genome (genomics) is transforming epidemiology, medicine and drug discovery (Palmer and Cardon, 2005, Ioannidis *et al.* 2006, Zheng *et al.* 2008, Saxena *et al.* 2007, WTCCC, 2007), and there is an ongoing refocusing of effort towards population-based genetic association studies for complex phenotypes (see Chapter Six). For many complex human conditions, the genetic basis of disease susceptibility, progression, severity and response to therapy has been increasingly emphasised in medical research. The ultimate goal of such research is the improvement of biological understanding, prevention, diagnostic tools and treatment (Davis and Khoury, 2006).

Completion of the human genome sequencing project was followed by three key advances that have created unprecedented opportunities for understanding the pathogenic basis of common human diseases: (1) Compilation of extensive catalogues of DNA sequence variants across the human genome ('polymorphic loci') (Frazer *et al.* 2007, Kruglyak, 2008, Manolio *et al.* 2008, Siva, 2008); (2) more rapid and cheaper molecular genetic technologies for evaluating common polymorphic sites; and (3) increasing availability of large, population-based human samples such as the European Prospective Investigation into Cancer and Nutrition (EPIC) (Gonzalez, 2006), the Framingham Heart Study (Jaquish, 2007) and the Avon Longitudinal Study of Parents and Children (ALSPAC) (Golding *et al.* 2001). The construction of large, national cohorts such as the UK Medical Research Council/Wellcome Trust Biobank (Palmer, 2007) has become appealing to funding bodies in many countries (Stafford, 2008, Burton *et al.* 2008), with planned or ongoing initiatives for national cohorts in a number of countries in Western Europe, Scandinavia, North America and Australasia (see Chapter Six). Although the genomics revolution and the generation of high-density single nucleotide polymorphism (SNP) maps has benefited the investigation of Mendelian diseases, our discussion will be restricted to common complex human conditions such as obesity, type 2 diabetes (T2D) and cardiovascular disease that are determined by multiple genetic and environmental factors. The major challenges facing most developed nations are those related to the rising number of cases, and in some instances prevalence, of common, complex diseases and the increasing complexity of their diagnosis, prevention and treatment (Zerhouni, 2003, and Chapter 7).

Given the rapidly changing nature of the field of genetic epidemiology, the large amounts of genomic data being generated at considerable cost to governments and corporations, and the apparent and the unforeseen obstacles facing progress, it is important to consider current initiatives in the context of expediting the discovery and characterisation of complex human disease genes. This chapter therefore reviews the state of knowledge about the human genome as related to SNPs and linkage disequilibrium (LD), discusses the potential applications of this knowledge to mapping complex disease genes using genome–wide association studies (GWASs), and finishes by describing some of the methodological and study design issues related to gene discovery. We have tried to summarise in this chapter the key current developments. However, the field of genetic epidemiology is evolving very rapidly and our knowledge base is currently expanding exponentially. It is therefore inevitable that we do not discuss here all of the applied and methodological work currently underway in association studies of complex human disease genetics in the current chapter.

Genomic information in mapping complex disease genes

The sequencing of the human genome remains the key enabling event in discovering regions of the genome involved in complex disease aetiology. However, the main focus of the human genome project was on a consensus human sequence, which by definition cannot contain information about individual differences of medical relevance (Cardon and Watkins, 2000). To make use of the consensus sequence, the SNP Consortium was formed in 1999, with other public and private projects, with the aim of discovering common polymorphism sites in the human genome (Sachidanandam *et al.* 2001). The burgeoning catalogue of common genetic variants that is being applied to association studies of complex phenotypes is a direct extension of the consortium's work. The natural next step in the SNP discovery phase was to genotype identified SNPs in specific individuals to begin to assess their potential usefulness for disease mapping (Kruglyak, 2008). The International HapMap Project (Conrad *et al.* 2006, Frazer *et al.* 2007), the first phase of which was completed in 2005, took this aim forward (Box 4.1. The logical successor to the HapMap project is to whole-genome sequence a larger number of genomes than the very small number involved in the initial Human Genome Project. Aided by the arrival of next-generation sequencing technologies that are much faster and cheaper than the traditional Sanger method, large-scale sequencing of thousands of human genomes is fast becoming reality (von Bubnoff, 2008). The recently initiated 1000 Genomes Project will involve sequencing the genomes of at least a thousand people from around the world over the next few years in order to provide much higher resolution data than the initial HapMap project (Siva, 2008, The 1000 Genomes Project) (Box 4.1).

The natural next stage in the progression from SNP genotyping has involved applications to gene discovery, reflecting the culmination of the first phase of the genomic framework studies (Box 4.1). An increasing number of genes associated with complex diseases (over 150 new validated genes since early 2007) have been discovered by association-based genetic mapping (Orr and Chanock, 2008). Genetic association studies are discussed in detail in Chapters One and Three.

Single nucleotide polymorphisms

Because of the low rate of mutation (around 10^{-8} per site per generation) compared with number of generations since the most recent common ancestor of any two humans (around 10^4 generations), most SNPs are thought to arise from a single historical mutational event. Across the human genome, there are far more SNPs than any other types of polymorphism (Wang *et al.* 1998) – at least 10 million SNPs in the human genome with frequency greater than 1%, yielding an average spacing of one every 290 base pairs (Kruglyak and Nickerson, 2001). Precise estimates of SNP frequencies are difficult to determine as allele frequency differences occur broadly throughout the genome, between populations and within many genes of known medical relevance (Slatkin, 2008).

There are four important advantages of using SNPs rather than other types of genetic polymorphism to investigate the genetic determinants of complex human diseases (Collins *et al.* 1998, Palmer and Cookson, 2001, Risch, 2000). First, SNPs are plentiful throughout the genome, being found in exons, introns, promoters,

Box 4.1: The International HapMap Project

This large project aimed to construct genome-wide maps of LD patterns in multiple populations (Gibbs *et al.* 2003). The project genotyped more than one SNP per 1,000 bp across the genome in samples from four human populations collected in the US, Nigeria, China and Japan. In validating such a broad spectrum of SNPs and in building these high-density maps, the HapMap project aims to facilitate genetic mapping across a broad array of complex phenotypes, including those relevant to diagnostic and therapeutic applications. Importantly, the raw data have been released publicly, allowing immediate use of the emerging maps by the scientific community. The project has also fostered development and application of various statistical methods for LD mapping.

The main practical objective of the HapMap project was to identify sets of SNPs that would take advantage of the LD patterns identified to allow more efficient genotyping (Gibbs *et al.* 2003). When LD is high, the redundancy between markers implies that most of the information can be captured without genotyping all markers. Non-redundant markers that capture most or all of the LD information in a given genomic region have been termed 'haplotype tagging' SNPs (Johnson *et al.* 2001, Goldstein *et al.* 2003a) or tag SNPs. Defining and genotyping a relatively small number of these SNPs allows unambiguous determination of the common haplotypes in a population and captures all or most of the LD within that region (Barrett and Cardon, 2006, Anderson *et al.* 2008). By this means, SNP-phenotype association studies can be done relatively efficiently, in contrast to genotyping all common variants in a given genomic region or in the entire genome (Zhang *et al.* 2008, Manolio *et al.* 2008). Recent data suggest that tagging SNPs identified by the HapMap project are broadly applicable to mapping common variants in many human populations (Conrad *et al.* 2006, De Bakker *et al.* 2006, Xing *et al.* 2008, Gu *et al.* 2008).

Phase 2 of the HapMap project was completed in 2007 and assayed over 3.1 million SNPs, covering 25-35% of common SNP variation in the four populations surveyed (Frazer *et al.* 2007). The current 1000 Genomes Project will extend the HapMap project further by sequencing the genomes of at least a thousand people from around the world over the next few years in order to provide much higher resolution data than the initial HapMap project (Siva, 2008, The 1000 Genomes Project).

methylation–related regulatory elements, microRNA interfering sites and loci, enhancers and intergenic regions, allowing them to be used as markers in dense positional cloning investigations using both randomly distributed markers and markers clustered within genes (Kruglyak, 1997, Collins *et al.* 1997). Furthermore, it is likely that alleles at some of these polymorphisms are themselves functional. Second, groups of adjacent SNPs may exhibit patterns of correlations that can be used to enhance gene mapping (as discussed in Box 4.1) (Nickerson *et al.* 1992) and that may highlight recombination 'hot spots' (Chakravarti, 1998). Third, inter-population differences in SNP frequencies can be used in population-based genetic studies (McKeigue, 1998, Kuhner *et al.* 2000). Fourth, SNPs are less mutable than other types of polymorphism (Stallings *et al.* 1991, Brookes, 1999) and this greater stability could allow more consistent estimates of gene-phenotype associations.

The common SNPs in the human genome have been subject to large cataloguing projects funded by both government and industry (Gray *et al.* 2000, Varmus, 2003, Reich *et al.* 2003). These efforts have involved targeted SNP discovery by mutation detection (Edwards and Bartlett, 2003) or primary resequencing in candidate genes or regions (Kruglyak and Nickerson, 2001, Carlson *et al.* 2003). As of late 2009, worldwide public efforts have identified more than 18 million SNPs, over 6.5 million of which have been validated (www.ncbi.nlm.nih.gov/SNP/index.html).

Many other SNPs present in major ethnic groups are likely to be discovered through increased efforts by industry and academic research groups, aided by improvements in DNA sequencing technology and capacity, and the increased availability of high-efficiency mutation scanning techniques. Although these enterprises have constructed large SNP databases that are constantly updated and growing rapidly (Box 4.2), this process is not yet complete. At present, the information contained in these databases is not infallible, as some of the putative polymorphisms are actually sequencing errors or rare or population-specific variants that are often not detected in subsequent studies. Despite the ever-increasing quantity and quality of information in SNP databases (Yang *et al.* 2008),

---

Box 4.2: Selected websites
SNP databases
- 1000 Genomes Project [www.1000genomes.org/page.php?page=home]
- dbSNP Polymorphism Repository [www.ncbi.nlm.nih.gov/SNP/]
- Cancer Genome Anatomy Project [http://cgap.nci.nih.gov/]
- Ensembl [www.ensembl.org/index.html]
- Génome Québec [www.genomequebec.com/index_e.asp]
- The Golden Path [http://genome.ucsc.edu]
- Human Genome Variation Database [http://hgvbase.cgb.ki.se/]
- The Human Genome Variation Society [www.genomic.unimelb.edu.au/mdi/]
- Human Gene Mutation Database [http://archive.uwcm.ac.uk/uwcm/mg/hgmd0.html]
- Human SNP Database [www-genome.wi.mit.edu/SNP/human/index.html]
- The International HapMap Project [www.hapmap.org/]
- LocusLink [www.ncbi.nih.gov/LocusLink/]
- NHLBI Programs for Genomic Applications Resources [http://pga.lbl.gov/PGA/PGA_inventory.html]
- OMIM – Online Mendelian Inheritance in Man™ [www.ncbi.nlm.nih.gov/entrez/query.fcgi?db=OMIM]
- SNP Consortium [http://snp.cshl.org/]
- SNP View [http://snp.gnf.org/]
- The Sanger Centre [www.sanger.ac.uk/]

Software
- An extensive list of genetic analysis software [http://linkage.rockefeller.edu/soft/list.html]

many investigators interested in further investigating genomic regions defined by GWASs, or in studying specific genes or pathways, continue to independently seek to identify sequence variants by primary resequencing in their own study populations (Yeager *et al.* 2008, Zheng *et al.* 2009), a practice that is likely to continue in the near to medium future.

In the context of medical research, SNPs have found widespread use in the delineation of genetic influences in multifactorial diseases such as breast cancer, cardiovascular disease, T2D and asthma, in attempts to fine map loci associated with complex human diseases, and as genetic markers to predict responses to drugs and adverse drug reactions (Nebert *et al.* 2008, Palmer and Cardon, 2005). There are at least seven primary areas of potential application for SNP technologies in improving our understanding of complex disease (Schork *et al.* 2000, Yamada, 2008, Manolio *et al.* 2008, Janssens and van Duijn, 2009, Khoury and Wacholder, 2009): (1) hypothesis-free gene discovery and mapping; (2) association-based candidate polymorphism testing; (3) pharmacogenetics; (4) diagnostics and risk profiling; (5) prediction of response to non-pharmacological environmental stimuli; (6) homogeneity testing and epidemiological study design; and (7) the definition of modifiable environmental aetiological factors using methods such as Mendelian randomisation (Ebrahim and Davey Smith, 2008) (see Chapter Seven). Given these possibilities, there have been dual imperatives to develop advanced technologies to detect and genotype SNPs for research and clinical applications (Box 4.2), and to concomitantly improve statistical approaches and study designs to allow SNP data to be incorporated into epidemiology and clinical medicine. Although in early stages of development and application, there is now also growing interest in the role of another form of common variation in the genome – copy-number variants (CNVs) – in human disease (McCarroll, 2008).

Linkage disequilibrium

Most SNPs lie outside genes and are not likely to alter gene structure or function in any way and therefore might not be directly associated with any change in phenotype (Collins *et al.* 1999). Thus, it is important to ascertain whether the DNA sequence variant under consideration is potentially directly functional (that is, could lead to the observed biology) or is indirectly correlated with another DNA sequence variant that is the actual cause of the phenotype of interest. Given that candidate genes are notoriously difficult to select (Cardon and Bell, 2001) and that functional data are rarely available for a given SNP, testing for indirect association is currently the operational paradigm within which most attempts at gene discovery are occurring. The concept of LD is discussed in other chapters. Loci in LD are generally in close physical proximity, but the actual distance (physical or genetic) varies dramatically (Figure 4.1b). When a variant is first introduced into a population by mutation, it will be perfectly correlated with nearby variants. Over successive generations meiotic recombination will break up the correlations among nearby variants, and LD will decay (Figure 4.1a). Indirect association

Figure 4.1: Theoretical (a) and observed (b) patterns of LD decay

Plotted using data from a chromosome-wide study of human chromosome 22 (Dawson *et al.* 2002). (a) The hypothetical decay in LD as function of recombination fraction between two loci. The three curves indicate different time-scales (numbers of generations) since the initial mutations that generated the markers. For two markers that recombine at rate θ, the correlation between them is reduced (by $1-\theta$) in each generation, so at generation t remaining disequilibrium is $E(D_t) = (1-\theta)^t$. (b) Decay trends in real data from chromosome 22. The general shape of theoretical decay is apparent in the empirical data, but there is a vast amount of variability so that knowing average decay gives little information about any specific pair of genetic loci.

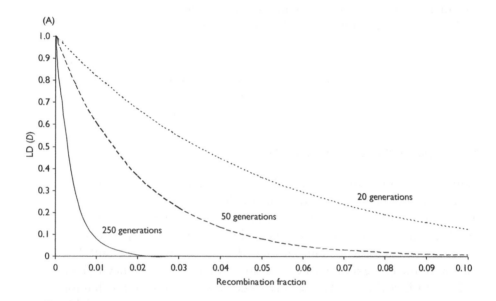

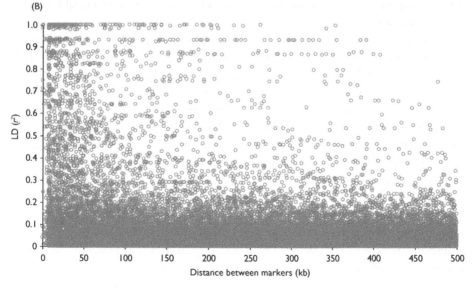

mapping relies on LD (allelic correlation) in the sense that the functional variant need not be studied at all, so long as one measures a variant that is in LD with it. LD patterns in the human genome have been the focus of intense research since the early 2000s because of the value of LD in localising disease–causing genes (Slatkin, 2008). Because of the extensive LD between neighbouring loci in the human genome, a subset of the SNPs in a region (tag SNPs) can be selected to capture most of the remaining common SNP variants (see also Chapter Three). Patterns of LD reveal the action of evolutionary processes and provide crucial information for association mapping of disease genes.

Many factors can influence LD, including genetic drift, population growth, admixture, population structure, natural selection, variable recombination and mutation rates, and gene conversion (Slatkin, 2008). The International HapMap Project was begun to describe disequilibrium patterns in some ethnic groups and has enabled the indirect association mapping of complex disease genes (The International HapMap Project, 2003, Frazer et al. 2007) (Box 4.1).

Haplotypes and haplotype estimation

Indirect association mapping by LD relies on gene–phenotype associations at the level of the population and requires a dense map of markers (Slatkin, 2008, Attia et al. 2009). LD mapping can be enhanced by examining multiple markers simultaneously or by using haplotypes, which are linear arrangements of closely linked alleles on the same chromosome that are inherited as a unit. Haplotype analysis in the context of disease association studies can be difficult (Toivonen et al. 2000, Attia et al. 2009), but haplotypes do contain at least as much information as the genotypes at each component locus, so they may prove essential for some disease gene studies.

For M biallelic markers there are 2^M possible haplotypes (though often many fewer are evident), and because we usually do not know in advance which haplotypes might be associated with disease, all are tested. Testing SNPs one at a time would require only M tests. In this regard, the greater information in haplotypes is offset by the cost of testing more of them. The growing use of phylogenetic and cladistic approaches derived from population genetics in human gene discovery investigations holds promise in this area (Templeton, 1996, Tachmazidou et al. 2007, Durrant et al. 2004), as they can assist in forming 'natural' groupings of haplotypes and thus reduce the degrees-of-freedom burden.

When LD is high, the redundancy among markers means that haplotypes can be used in association studies to efficiently map common alleles that might influence the susceptibility to common diseases, as well as for reconstructing genomic evolution (Slatkin, 2008). When LD is low, haplotypes will generally be useful in refining SNP-phenotype associations only if they help delineate rare allele frequencies or if there are significant interactions among the SNPs in their effect on the trait, in other words if there is epistatic interaction. In complex diseases, where multiple variant loci contribute to disease susceptibility, haplotypes are therefore also potentially important because different combinations of particular alleles in the same gene may act as a 'meta-allele' or 'meta-SNP' and have different effects on the protein product and on transcriptional regulation (Mira *et al.* 2004, Chen *et al.* 2009).

In population-based studies using unrelated individuals, the parental origin of each allele of a genotype is not known (so-called 'phase unknown' status); haplotypes for double heterozygotes are uncertain and must be estimated (Thomas *et al.* 2004). Statistical methods and software are available to estimate haplotypes from phase unknown genotype data in large population-based samples of unrelated individuals or in family data (Thomas *et al.* 2004, Schaid, 2002, Abecasis *et al.* 2000, Niu *et al.* 2002, Stephens *et al.* 2001, Excoffier and Slatkin, 1995). Maximum-likelihood methods have been developed to enable the testing of statistical association between haplotypes and a wide variety of traits, including binary, ordinal and quantitative traits (Schaid *et al.* 2002, Sham *et al.* 2004). However, the use of haplotypes derived from phase-unknown genotype data is not always straightforward, and the ultimate value of these techniques for gene mapping is not yet clear (Liu *et al.* 2008).

Despite a dip in interest in gene mapping using haplotyping during the GWAS era, there has been a recent resurgence of interest in investigating haplotypes spurred on by the promise of very high-density data from new whole-genome sequencing projects, such as the 1000 genomes project, and from new and sophisticated approaches to haplotyping, such as Bayesian partition models that exploit evolutionary information (Tachmazidou *et al.* 2007). Current imputation techniques used for GWAS marker panels rely on LD properties and have also resulted in renewed interest in haplotype-based methods (Browning, 2008).

LD patterns across the genome

The availability of dense sets of SNPs together with improved genotyping technology and statistical methods were necessary developments to enable gene discovery by indirect association analysis. However, more information regarding the architecture of the genome was required to map genes efficiently. The extreme variability in the correlation between physical distance and LD in a given genomic region (Figure 4.1) means that two genetic variants that are physically close will sometimes be completely independent, whereas loci that are very far apart will sometimes be highly correlated. Thus, when LD is low, screening nearly all of the SNPs in a given region could still miss the relevant locus. When LD is high, evidence for association can be found for most of the loci examined, thereby rendering the experiment inefficient and yielding little information about the precise localisation of the aetiological variant (Lawrence *et al.* 2005). These two extremes are depicted in Figure 4.2, where a chromosome region in which many markers are associated with the outcome (Figure 4.2a) is contrasted with a region in which only a single marker reveals evidence for association (Figure 4.2b). The different patterns of disease association are due to different LD patterns in the chromosome regions (Figure 4.2c).

Until the mid–2000s, little was known about LD patterns in the genome except for a few well characterised genes and gene families. However, studies of large genomic regions, entire chromosomes and the entire genome have now added to this knowledge base, highlighting the importance of dense marker panels

Figure 4.2: The role of LD in facilitating allelic association

(4.2a and 4.2b): disease association profiles for a hypothetical disease in which the aetiological locus confers an odds ratio of 3.0. Markers in (a) show extensive background LD, so many are associated with trait. Markers in (b) show little LD, so only the causal locus is associated. The distribution of LD for these two scenarios shown in (c) to illustrate that knowing local patterns can help to delineate the expected patterns of association and design efficient novel studies. Data are taken from chromosome 22 (Dawson *et al.* 2002) in which an arbitrary locus was designated the disease gene in high and low LD regions of the chromosome. The decay in odds ratio was computed as described by Zondervan and Cardon (2004).

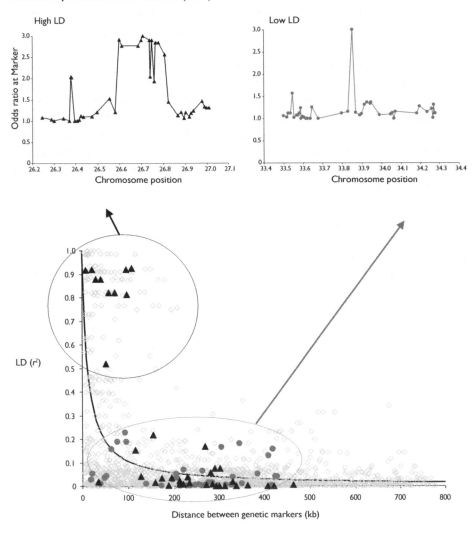

and revealing extensive variability in LD patterns and recombination rates (The International HapMap Project, 2005, Barrett and Cardon, 2006, Frazer *et al.* 2007, Slatkin, 2008). The International HapMap Project was undertaken in recognition of the need for further information to enable appropriate study design and more accurate interpretation of association studies (Box 4.1).

Genome-wide association studies

Recently, human genome epidemiology has had unprecedented success in discovering validated genes underlying common, complex diseases by undertaking GWASs of large population-based samples (WTCCC, 2007, Kruglyak, 2008). There are various approaches available to investigate the relationship between genetic variants and specific disease phenotypes, including linkage and candidate gene approaches. Each approach has important strengths and limitations (Palmer and Cardon, 2005). Both linkage and candidate gene approaches have generally failed to discover replicable genetic associations with common, chronic disease phenotypes (Slatkin, 2008, Clarke *et al.* 2007, Chanock *et al.* 2007, Colhoun *et al.* 2003). In contrast, GWASs provide an unbiased approach to identify genomic regions (coding and non-coding sequences) containing genetic variants causally associated with disease phenotypes (WTCCC, 2007) (Box 4.3). The current focus

---

Box 4.3: An example of the application of a genome-wide association study

Recent examination of genome-wide data has revealed an important example of how a non-hypothesis-driven application of genetic analysis on a genome-wide scale can reveal novel pathways with confirmed association with complex disease phenotypes. Analysis of the Wellcome Trust Case Control Study type 2 diabetes (T2D) data (based on 1,924 cases and 2,938 non-matched, general population ('universal') controls) generated strong evidence for the association of variation in a region of chromosome 16 with disease risk (WTCCC, 2007, Zeggini *et al.* 2007). Further analysis taking into account informative heterogeneity in this signal and the potential co-association of body mass index and T2D then led to the finding that the effect observed with T2D (around a 40% elevation in the odds of disease) was entirely driven by an association of this genetic variation with elevated fat mass. In a follow-up replication study of approximately 37,000 individuals, this fat mass association has been shown to related to an increase of approximately 7% and 15% in the case of fat mass (measured using dual-energy X-ray absorptiometry, DXA) as a result of the carriage of one or two risk alleles at this locus, respectively. In terms of obesity, this variation yields an odds ratio of approximately 1.7, equating to an approximately 70% elevation in the odds of obesity if there are two predisposing alleles (Frayling *et al.* 2007). The gene implicated by the location of this variation is now known to be the renamed 'fat mass and obesity associated gene' (*FTO*). This is the first confirmed association of common genetic variation with obesity and heralds a paradigm shift in the strategy used for the identification of genetic variation involved in the aetiology of common conditions. By enabling hypothesis-free research, the GWAS approach has evolved as a powerful new way to understand complex disease biology.

on GWASs has stemmed partly from the realisation that candidate-gene association studies of complex phenotypes often either fail to discover susceptibility loci or produce results that are not themselves reproducible in replication studies (Clarke *et al.* 2007, Chanock *et al.* 2007).

What is a 'genome-wide' association study?

Although 'genome-wide' implies complete coverage, not all such analyses are the same and they are not always directly comparable (without imputation, using linkage disequilibrium and HapMap data). For example, marker panels of 500,000 or more SNPs are now commercially available as 'whole-genome' panels. In constructing such panels, one could select 500,000 or more SNPs in a variety of ways, such as by focusing only on genes or on putatively functional variants, by using LD tagging or by using SNPs that are randomly distributed throughout the genome (Barrett and Cardon, 2006). None of the currently available marker panels covers all variation in the genome, so by a strict definition none offers a genome-wide study. Although most GWAS panels of SNPs provide substantial coverage of common variation in non-African populations, the precise extent is strongly dependent on the frequencies of alleles of interest and on specific considerations of study design (Barrett and Cardon, 2006). Overall, despite substantial differences in genotyping technologies, marker selection strategies and number of markers assayed, the first-generation high-throughput platforms all offered similar levels of genome coverage – less than 80% of the common genetic variants in most populations (Barrett and Cardon, 2006) (a figure that, in practical terms, will equate to a realised coverage of around 60-70% after quality control measures are in place). Coverage has now improved with denser panels; imputation of markers using HapMap data can also increase coverage (Anderson *et al.* 2008). GWASs will therefore continue to require qualifiers describing their aims, assumptions and presumed coverage. The concern is not so much that what they do find will be false, but rather how many and what sort of genetic variants they will miss (Kruglyak, 2008, Anderson *et al.* 2008).

Complete resequencing of the entire genomes (or even just the 'exome', i.e. all the exons) of case and control individuals would be ideal, but this technology is only just becoming fully available and affordable (Siva, 2008, Hoggart *et al.* 2008b). The high-density marker panels used by the International HapMap Project (Box 4.1) and in industry offer the most immediate form of genome-wide coverage. Although rare variants are under-represented, as much as 85-90% of the genetic variants that are common in the populations evaluated are currently available.

Reducing the genotyping burden

The growing density of SNP maps together with the growing availability of large case series and cohort studies have made GWASs feasible for all but the rarest complex diseases. However, despite the dramatic drop in genotyping costs that, for some technologies, have realised the goal of <US$0.001 per genotype (a target once regarded as highly ambitious), testing all of the estimated 10 million common SNPs would currently cost at least US$10,000 per individual, or US$20 million for a single study of 1,000 cases and controls. Exhaustive genotyping for association is thus currently impractical.

There are at least two strategies for reducing the number of SNPs that need to be genotyped (Collins *et al.* 1997) – one based on direct association and the genotyping of all potentially functional SNPs across the genome ('sequence-based') (Peltonen and McKusick, 2001, Botstein and Risch, 2003) and the other based on indirect association and LD-tagging SNPs across the genome ('map-based').

The sequence-based approach makes savings by assuming that some variants are more likely to influence complex traits than others. Prioritised lists of such variants can be compiled (Risch, 2000, Botstein and Risch, 2003) that decrease the number of SNPs to 50,000-100,000. However, despite the availability of over 18 million SNPs in public databases, further work may be needed to identify all SNPs at the top of the priority list (for example, non-synonymous, non-conservative coding changes (Risch, 2000)). In addition, many coding changes are rarer in their allele frequencies than non-coding changes, thus creating sample size challenges unless the genes have large effects. This approach was trialled in the WTCCC by undertaking a study of about 14,500 non-synonymous SNPs (nsSNPs) across four case-control studies – ankylosing spondylitis, autoimmune thyroid disease, multiple sclerosis and breast cancer (Burton *et al.* 2007). Although the study successfully identified two new non-synonymous variants contributing to ankylosing spondylitis susceptibility, it has become clear that little advantage is offered by this study design given the ever-decreasing costs of a genome scan of 500,000 or more tagging or randomly selected SNPs. The majority of the nsSNPs investigated in the WTCCC study (Burton *et al.* 2007) are captured by one or more SNPs in current GWAS panels (Evans *et al.* 2008). Information from commercially available nsSNP panels is therefore largely redundant with 'full' GWAS panels. Although specialised nsSNP panels will capture rare variants better than more generalised GWAS panels, current GWAS sample sizes preclude detection of rare SNPs in association analyses unless they have moderate to large effects (Evans *et al.* 2008).

The map-based approach is the current operational paradigm for GWAS-based gene discovery in complex disease. This approach makes no assumptions about the genes involved or the type of the mutation, although it does assume that disease alleles or haplotypes are sufficiently frequent to have been captured by the original tagging study. This approach is unlikely to capture rare variants (see later).

One approach that can reduce genotyping requirements under both the map-based or sequence-based strategies is the use of 'generic' or 'universal' controls. The use of 'universal' general population controls is a powerful strategy for gene discovery (WTCCC, 2007) in GWASs, and is increasingly being used worldwide. Genome-wide SNP data from many studies have been made publicly available at the urging of funding bodies and scientific journals. These data have many potential uses, including the concept of 'universal controls', where a set of control samples genotyped for one project can be used to increase power or decrease cost for future projects. This hypothesis was tested (and verified) in two ways as part of the Wellcome Trust Case Control Consortium (WTCCC, 2007): (1) the project used controls ascertained in markedly different ways (the 1958 British Birth Cohort and randomly selected blood donors from the UK Blood Service) and observed very few meaningful differences in allele frequencies between the two groups; and (2) the project successfully used this combined set of controls to test for association with seven distinct case groups, identifying more than 20 subsequently verified associations. Given that these controls have similar ancestry to the many European samples in other countries, it is likely that they can be safely incorporated into further GWAS projects with careful attention to data annotation and curation. The potential use of common control groups within genetic epidemiological studies is certainly greater than it is within conventional risk-factor epidemiology. This is because the low level of confounding that exists between genetic variants and a wide range of socioeconomic, behavioural and physiological risk factors means that non-random or matched selection of a control group will not, in general, generate differences in allele frequency (beyond that produced by population stratification), whereas such selection will produce control groups that differ markedly in terms of non-genetic factors (Davey Smith *et al.* 2007). One likely role for large cohort initiatives such as UK Biobank will be to provide further universal controls (see Chapter Six).

A potential issue related to the use of general population samples as control groups is that these samples will almost certainly be 'contaminated' with individuals with either undiagnosed or latent disease. The effects on statistical power of phenotype error, also known as diagnostic error, have been quantified (Edwards *et al.* 2005, Zheng and Tian, 2005). Although random errors in phenotype classification should not affect the type 1 error rate of genetic case control studies (Edwards *et al.* 2005), any misclassification will reduce real differences between the groups and hence the power to detect genetic association (Mote and Anderson, 1965). The work of Zheng and Tian (Zheng and Tian, 2005) indicated that, for prevalent diseases (prevalence $\geq 10\%$), when individuals were diagnosed with 95% sensitivity and 95% specificity, the required sample size almost doubled compared with the situation in which cases and controls were correctly identified. However, the effect of misclassifying an affected individual as unaffected on the statistical power of the test is not the same as the reverse error, and the impact of each depends on the prevalence of disease (Edwards *et al.* 2005). For example, as prevalence of diseases approaches zero, the cost of misclassifying a control as a case becomes infinitely large, whereas penalty for misclassifying an affected individual as unaffected approaches zero (Edwards *et al.* 2005). For most diseases for which prevalence is ≤10%, it is more important to ensure that cases are truly affected rather than ensuring that controls are really unaffected (Edwards *et al.* 2005).

Fine mapping through the assessment of all (including rare) variation and localisation of association signals remain issues for GWASs – what is being 'discovered' is not necessarily the functional genes themselves, but robustly replicable statistical associations, which may well occur in nearby loci (Saccone *et al.* 2008). There are now several examples of validated genetic signals in specific genes initially discovered in GWASs for which the functional variant(s) have subsequently been found in nearby genes (Loos *et al.* 2008) (Box 4.3). For example, in the region containing the haematopoietically expressed homeobox (*HHEX*) and insulin degrading enzyme (*IDE*) genes, strong linkage disequilibrium extends across three genes, two of which are plausible candidates (Zeggini *et al.* 2007, Saxena *et al.* 2007). The functional variant might also not lie anywhere near the coding parts of a gene, but might instead influence a regulatory element that might or might not yet be characterised. The *CDKN2A–CDKN2B* locus, which contains cyclin-dependent kinase inhibitor genes, seems to be an example of this: the maximum statistical ssociation is some distance from the nearest genes (Zeggini *et al.* 2007, Saxena *et al.* 2007).

Putting the pieces together: methodological and study design issues

Until recently, the ability to undertake adequate genetic association studies (adequate in the sense that they are able to provide clear evidence that a particular gene is or is not implicated in disease susceptibility) has been seriously compromised by: (1) use of sample sizes too small for the identification of variants with plausible effect sizes (with ORs ≤ 1.2); (2) difficulties choosing candidate genes with reasonable prior odds for an important effect; (3) the logistics and expense associated with generating a comprehensive survey of genetic variation in a chosen gene; (4) poor understanding of the patterns of LD in the human genome; and (5) lack of progress in understanding which non-coding regions are likely to be functionally important. These problems are now resolvable for many diseases for the following reasons:

- **Large, extensively characterised studies**. Large, homogenous case-control and cohort studies are available, providing excellent power to detect relatively modest genetic effects;
- **Availability of replication samples**. A growing ethos of collaboration and intellectual generosity in genetic epidemiology has resulted in the formation of large multinational consortia (some with over 100,000 subjects) allowing the extensive cross-replication and meta-analyses of findings across multiple large studies;

- **High-throughput genotyping platforms.** High-throughput platforms have steadily increased in accuracy and efficiency; genotyping costs have recently reduced to below $0.001 per SNP genotype (Steemers and Gunderson, 2007);
- **Proof of principle that GWASs can discover common genes of modest effect.** GWASs of large, population-based samples investigating complex diseases have discovered over 150 validated genes in the past 24 months (Orr and Chanock, 2008); and
- **Improved biostatistical and bioinformatic tools.** We have new approaches and tools available to us, and we benefit from the increasing transfer of technology from other areas of mathematics and statistics into genetic epidemiology (Sieberts and Schadt, 2007, Zhu *et al.* 2008, Schadt *et al.* 2008). These new tools are greatly enhancing our capacity to discover important aetiological genetic variants and gene-environment associations.

Increasingly complete SNP databases, better genotyping, high-density LD maps and large population samples are essential for complex trait association studies, but they do not guarantee success. Other obstacles remain, many of which are outside the investigator's control. Examples, reviewed elsewhere, include technical issues in genotyping, limitations to our understanding of LD (Orr and Chanock, 2008, Slatkin, 2008) and difficulties in investigating gene-phenotype associations involving multiple interacting genetic and environmental factors (Janssens and van Duijn, 2009, Khoury and Wacholder, 2009). We will not address these issues again here, but will instead highlight some additional factors emerging from the ongoing integration of the large-scale genetic and epidemiological data.

Statistical methods

The focus on SNP genotyping has made it clear that concomitant statistical advances in the use of LD in mapping complex trait genes will also be required (Slatkin, 2008, Janssens and van Duijn, 2009, Khoury and Wacholder, 2009). Optimal strategies for the application of SNPs and LD mapping to both gene discovery and gene characterisation (especially in terms of gene-gene and gene-environment interaction) in common diseases remain unclear, and an ongoing broad re-examination of mapping methodologies and study designs has been underway for the past decade (Slatkin, 2008, Janssens and van Duijn, 2009, Khoury and Wacholder, 2009). The required methodological development in genetic statistics is non-trivial given the high-dimensional data being produced and the underlying biological complexity of common human diseases.

The scarcity of sophisticated statistical techniques to deal with the complicated problems inherent in genetic investigations of complex diseases is currently a critical factor limiting the ultimate success of human complex disease gene discovery and utilisation programs (Palmer and Cardon, 2005, Kanehisa and Bork, 2003, Wolfe and Li, 2003) – in terms of both discovery and translation. This remains a bottleneck for the utilisation of large-scale population-based resources for genetic epidemiological and genomic research, particularly as newly discovered genes are now being characterised in the context of richly phenotyped longitudinal cohort studies (Frayling *et al.* 2007). Statistical genetics and bioinformatics are key enabling technological endeavours internationally, and so far research capacity in these areas has lagged seriously behind our technical ability to general large amounts of genomic data.

One practical challenge facing the use of tagging SNPs concerns the definition of the genomic region to be tagged. Tagging was initially described as a means of efficiently genotyping (Johnson *et al.* 2001) but was later joined to the notion of haplotype blocks, which are regions of very high LD separated by regions of low LD (Daly *et al.* 2001, Gabriel *et al.* 2002, Cardon and Abecasis, 2003). As block boundaries are not always consistent within or between populations (Ke *et al.* 2004, Crawford *et al.* 2004) or between statistical definitions of them (Schulze *et al.* 2004), it is not yet clear that block tags defined in one sample will capture the same information in another. Ultimately, the region-definition problem could be addressed empirically by examining multiple samples drawn from many populations, or theoretically by statistical methods that retain the efficiencies of high LD yet relax the dependence on physical boundaries of the region studied (Carlson *et al.* 2004). With respect to the application of these techniques to the analysis of disease association, these issues become of great importance. Although allelic association may have a precise genomic location (often determined by the machinery of genotyping), the presence of this within a block of LD will essentially define the window of interest with regard to further investigation. The definition of this window (be it by patterns of recombination or nomenclature/annotation) at this point becomes a critical element in the full elucidation of the role of a particular genomic region in disease. This has been an important consideration in the design of follow-up studies to initial GWASs.

Missing data, an issue for genetic analysis generally, are a particular problem for LD-tagging and haplotypic analysis. Sequencing or genotyping a given set of SNPs is rarely 100% complete; in the absence of strong LD, this can lead to a cumulative problem with missing data, with each additional SNP included in a haplotypic analysis or imputation analysis. Other fields of statistical investigation have learned that simply ignoring missing data or restricting analysis to individuals with complete data can lead to biased or inefficient analyses (Little and Yau, 1996, Verbeke and Molenberghs, 2000, Molenberghs *et al.* 2002, Mallinckrodt *et al.* 2003, Raghunathan, 2004, White *et al.* 2003). This problem worsens if data are not missing at random, as may be the case with systematic errors in genotyping assays. Methods for dealing appropriately with missing data, largely related to imputation, are available but have only begun to be applied to genetic epidemiology relatively recently (Browning, 2008, Balding, 2006). There is thus a need for further research on the extent to which missing data are a problem in genetic association analyses of SNPs and haplotypes, and on the application of methods for dealing appropriately with missing data in genetic association studies.

High-dimensional data and systems biology

The fundamental issue of how to deal with the sheer volume of genetic data being produced has only just begun to be addressed. Although the initial wave of GWASs focused on relatively simple case-control designs and dichotomous phenotypes, the focus is increasingly on complex quantitative traits and longitudinal data. High-dimensional data often exists at two levels – genomic (genotype) and phenotype. For instance, the authors of this chapter, with others, are currently undertaking both GWASs (>500,000 SNPs) and candidate gene 'pathway' analyses of complex phenotypes and trajectories in the ALPSAC (Ness, 2004) and Raine (Huang *et al.* 2006) Birth Cohorts. These are richly phenotyped cohort studies, and each has over 10,000 variables measured for each participant, assessed throughout early life and childhood from before birth to age 18. These studies are likely to implicate a large number of SNPs clustered within genes that may interact with each other to influence pathogenic pathways in the context of a large number of highly correlated phenotypes.

Modelling networks of genes and higher order gene-gene and gene-environment interactions will become increasingly important in light of the assessment of both more complex phenotypes and more complex types of genetic variation (such as copy-number variants, which may need to be analysed as continuously varying entities). One aspect of methodological work will thus be to develop optimal methods to investigate higher-order interactions among genetic variants and environmental factors (Hahn *et al.* 2003, Ritchie *et al.* 2001, Hunter, 2005, Evans *et al.* 2006). For instance, previous work has developed logistic regression methods for GWASs that model gene-gene and gene-environment interaction; simulation studies have demonstrated that for many genetic models this approach is more powerful than marker-by-marker analysis, even allowing for the need to correct for the number of analyses performed (Evans *et al.* 2006).

There are two primary ways to deal with the issues related to high-dimensional data: (1) interpreting the findings in high dimensionality human data by integrating other types of data and networks from other systems (Schadt *et al.* 2008, Keller *et al.* 2008, Feinendegen *et al.* 2008, Farber *et al.* 2008); and (2) integrating data more formally to build mathematical models (networks) that infer relationships among variables of interest (Zhu *et al.* 2008, Chen *et al.* 2008). A further potential approach to high-dimensional data has already been exploited for the analysis of genotypic data. In efforts to resolve latent structure within genetic data attributable to population ancestry, principal components methods have been applied to GWAS data (Price *et al.* 2006, Li and Yu, 2007). These approaches need not be limited to genotypic data alone. The application of similar techniques to the simultaneous analysis of both complex patterns of genomic variation and complex phenotypes may represent a promising future approach to high-dimensional datasets.

Returning to the question of biological involvement, a challenge in the post-genome era is deciphering the possible function of individual genes and gene networks that drive disease. Genetic variation in complex phenotypes can be viewed as perturbations to an entire biological system, and these perturbations can be viewed as resulting in changes in genomic or transcriptional networks, ultimately altering the susceptibility to a complex disease or condition (Schadt, 2006). It is becoming increasingly clear that the mechanisms governing common, complex conditions are likely to encompass numerous factors from multiple biological systems, which need to be studied at the systems level (Keller *et al.* 2008, Feinendegen *et al.* 2008, Farber *et al.* 2008, Zhu *et al.* 2008) in addition to studying the function of a single gene or even a pathway to which a gene belongs. In particular, the use of Bayesian network methods to integrate many different types of data, including genotype, expression, DNA-protein binding and protein-protein interaction, appear very promising (Sieberts and Schadt, 2007, Zhu *et al.* 2007).

Emerging network approaches, aimed at processing high-dimensional biological data by integrating data from multiple sources, are some of the first applications of statistical genetics to identify multiple genetic perturbations that alter the states of molecular networks and that in turn push systems into disease states. Evolving statistical procedures that operate on networks will be critical to extracting information related to complex phenotypes such as disease, as research goes beyond a single-gene focus.

Power, *p*-values and multiple testing

Growing experience with complex disease genetics has made clear the need to reduce both type 1 and type 2 error (Lander and Kruglyak, 1995, Risch, 2000, Cardon and Bell, 2001, Colhoun *et al.* 2003). Power for studies of allelic association will depend primarily on sample size, the effect size of the susceptibility locus, the strength of LD with a marker, the frequencies of susceptibility and marker alleles, and the number of markers tested (Zondervan and Cardon, 2004). Simple power calculations for a representative GWAS of 2,000 cases and 2,000 controls (around the median sample size for current GWASs) are shown in Figure 4.3. For simplicity, power calculations assume a SNP of log-additive (for a binary outcome) or additive (for a continuous outcome) effect and make similar assumptions regarding an appropriate genome-wide significance threshold to those made by the Wellcome Trust Case Control Consortium (WTCCC, 2007). Power estimates were produced using the program QUANTO (Gauderman and Morrison, 2006) for a range of minor allele frequencies (MAFs) and for an overall α of $p = 5 \times 10^{-7}$, and $R^2 = 1$ between marker and trait loci (Figure 4.3). Simple power calculations for presence or absence of the disease suggest that overall study power is high enough to detect an OR of at least 1.5 for SNPs with a MAF of at least 10% (Figure 4.3a) Such a study design would be associated with >80% power to detect OR $\geq$ 1.35 for SNPs $\geq$ 20% MAF.

Simple power calculations for GWAS analyses within the case group are based on the association of SNP genotype with a continuous phenotype. The overall study power is high enough to detect genes explaining $\geq$0.25 SD of a quantitative

Figure 4.3: Sample size estimates for case-control analyses of SNPs

(4.3a and 4.3b): Power calculations for case-control status in 2,000 cases and 2,000 controls (4.3a) or for a normally distributed quantitative trait in 2,000 cases (4.3b) for a range of minor allele frequencies (MAFs). Calculations assume a SNP of log-additive or additive effect, an overall α of $p = 5 \times 10^{-7}$, and $R^2 = 1$ between markers and quantitative-phenotype-associated alleles.

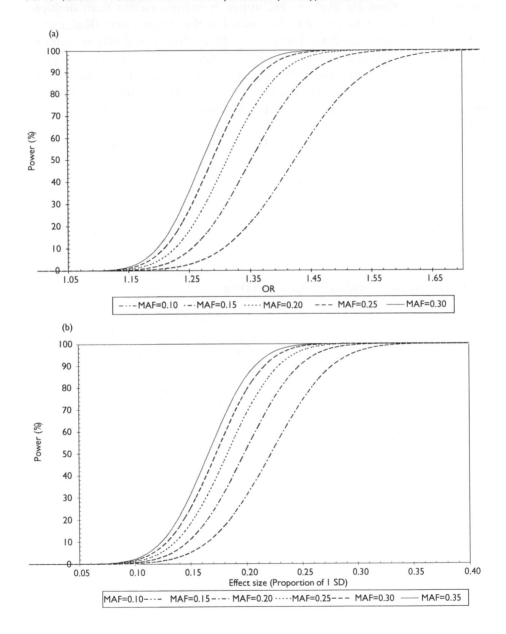

trait with MAF ≥ 0.15 (Figure 4.3b). Framed independently of allele frequency, this study would have >80% power to detect an additive genetic main effect explaining $\geq 1.5\%$ of total phenotypic variance in a quantitative trait. Thus, at a stringent α, such a study design would have good power for its primary aim to detect genes of fairly modest effect sizes on disease risk or on disease-related quantitative traits. However, rarer SNPs will lead to the need for very large (in some cases logistically improbable) sample sizes (Figure 4.3). This emphasises the recognition that genetic association studies have been generally underpowered until relatively recently (Cardon and Palmer, 2003, Colhoun *et al.* 2003, Orr and Chanock, 2008), and that even larger studies will be required in future in order to detect rarer alleles or loci and interactions of very modest effect. Very large and extensively characterised cohort studies will be needed not only for discovery, but also for the subsequent characterisation of discovered variants (see Chapter Six). Testing of large numbers of SNPs for association with one or more traits raises important statistical issues about false-positive rates and levels of statistical significance (Risch and Merikangas, 1996). Although the application of crude analyses and extensive replication of grossly associated variants from genome-wide analyses can yield robust associations (Frayling *et al.* 2007, Scuteri *et al.* 2007), an inevitable exploration of smaller effect sizes and more questionable associations require comprehensive assessment. Post hoc corrections tend to be too conservative, especially given that many (such as a simple Bonferroni correction (Rosner, 1990)) do not take proper account of the correlation between SNPs in LD with each other. Tagged SNPs have a special relationship in this regard. As the objective of tagging is to minimise redundancy in order to gain efficiency, tagged SNPs are chosen to be as independent as possible. Use of tag SNPs therefore requires more stringent correction than studies of the same number of correlated genomic SNPs. With correlated markers, statistical techniques to correct for multiple comparisons are emerging (Ziegler *et al.* 2008, Rice *et al.* 2008, Moskvina and Schmidt, 2008, Hoggart *et al.* 2008a), but replication of genetic association findings in independent population samples remains the gold standard for complex disease genetics (Chanock *et al.* 2007, Clarke *et al.* 2007) (see Replication section, p 116).

Population heterogeneity

Population heterogeneity is a potentially serious issue for gene discovery in any population-based study of complex diseases (Risch *et al.* 2002, Cardon and Palmer, 2003, Feldman *et al.* 2003, Shifman *et al.* 2003, Freedman *et al.* 2004, Marchini *et al.* 2004a). Disease prevalence often changes with geography and ethnicity, and allele frequencies can vary widely throughout the world (Cavalli-Sforza *et al.* 1994). In addition, there is likely to be a high degree of variation in LD between populations of different origins (Zavattari *et al.* 2000, Shifman *et al.* 2003) and between different genomic regions (Watkins *et al.* 1994, Jorde *et al.* 1994, Dawson *et al.* 2002, Patil *et al.* 2001, Phillips *et al.* 2003), leading to differences in genetic-physical map correlations, estimates of LD and haplotypes, tagging SNP selections and other outcomes. This heterogeneity can complicate or even prevent gene discovery and cloud apparent evidence for replication.

For both candidate gene and GWASs of many complex diseases, case–control designs have become the approach of choice. A major criticism of such studies in the past has been potentially undetected population stratification: spurious association may arise or true associations may be masked when allelic frequencies vary across subpopulations (for example, subjects from different ethnic groups (Ewens and Spielman, 1995)). This is a potential issue for both direct candidate gene approaches and indirect, LD-based association (Jorde, 2000). Such stratification may result from recent admixture or from poorly matched cases and controls.

Research on the potential effects of population stratification in large samples has been spurred on by the creation of large, population-based cohorts such as UK BioBank (Marchini *et al.* 2004a, Freedman *et al.* 2004, Palmer, 2007). Early studies examined the performance of genomic control under the promising scenarios of large samples and found that the larger the sample size, the larger the potential biasing effect of stratification (Marchini *et al.* 2004a, Freedman *et al.* 2004). It became clear that we may need to type many hundreds or even thousands of markers to detect and control subtle stratification in large samples, as slight levels of population structure become increasingly important with larger sample sizes (Marchini *et al.* 2004a). Fortunately, dense genotyping has occurred anyway as part of current GWASs. The adoption and widespread use of genomic control is particularly important at the moment, given the level of activity in the construction of large 'biobanks' throughout the world (see Chapter Six). Efforts to deal with substructure have focused on the use of multivariate statistical modelling applied to GWAS data (WTCCC, 2007) or on the use of a smaller number of ancestry-informative markers within and between populations (Salari *et al.* 2005). Given that only 10–15% of human genetic variation is predicted to be due to between-population differences (Shriver *et al.* 1997, Barbujani *et al.* 1997), and that a fraction (2–12%) of SNPs are more informative than the median microsatellite (in terms of informativeness) (Rosenberg *et al.* 2003), current work is aimed at exploiting both genetic and demographic data, where available, in efforts to account for hidden population structure.

Direct estimation of the degree of potential inflation of association test statistics using dense panels of SNPs ('genomic control') (Satten *et al.* 2001, Devlin *et al.* 2001b, Devlin *et al.* 2001a, Overall and Nichols, 2001, Bacanu *et al.* 2002, Pritchard and Rosenberg, 1999, Pritchard *et al.* 2000, Marchini *et al.* 2004b, Freedman *et al.* 2004), coupled with well designed, well conducted and appropriately analysed and interpreted population-based studies of unrelated controls, has greatly reduced the potential for confounding by population stratification (Cardon and Palmer, 2003). Statistical methods have been developed to detect and correct for substructure and are largely based around principal component analysis, such as the program Eigenstrat (Price *et al.* 2006, Li and Yu, 2007).

Explorations of genome-wide data have suggested that population substructure can generally be dealt with. The Wellcome Trust Case Control Consortium (WTCCC, 2007) demonstrated the ability of dense SNP data typed as part of a GWAS panel to detect fine-scale population stratification within a homogeneous population of cases and controls for seven diseases in UK-based populations. The vast majority of loci investigated by the WTCCC showed no evidence of stratification or recent selection (WTCCC, 2007). The few loci exhibiting such stratification were easily identified and removed. The availability of ancestry-informative markers within GWAS marker panels and statistical methods to analyse and correct for substructure (Price *et al.* 2006, Li and Yu, 2007) mean that substructure has generally not been a major issue in current gene discovery projects. However, the GWASs conducted to date have been heavily weighted towards population samples from northern Europe.

Because almost all of the GWASs undertaken to date have made use of cases and controls exclusively from populations of northern European ancestry, little is known about the frequency of risk alleles in other populations. The 'transferability' of LD patterns derived from HapMap data, and hence of tag SNPs selected using these data, across multiple ethnic groups or populations has been the subject of multiple investigations (Xing *et al.* 2008, Slatkin, 2008). Many ongoing and forthcoming GWASs rely critically on the validity and practical feasibility of using a universal core set of tag SNPs. In general, tag SNPs appear to be broadly transferrable across populations, but there are some notable exceptions (Gu *et al.* 2008). As we move away from 'Eurocentric' studies to investigate other ethnic groups, the issue of trans-population generalisability will become an increasingly important area of research (Slatkin, 2008, Hu *et al.* 2008, Angius *et al.* 2008, Cooper *et al.* 2008). An initial study investigating validated SNPs derived from GWASs across 53 different populations found that, although not large enough to indicate the possibility of selection occurring at functional loci, variation in risk allele frequencies between populations does exist and may contribute to differences in trait or locus association between human populations (Myles *et al.* 2008). Although such data are being explored further, more examples of GWASs in differing populations are still required to assess the extent to which differences in population-specific genomic architecture influence realised phenotypes. Many modern urban populations are likely to exhibit both known and cryptic substructure across groups, as well as admixture within individuals. Great care will need to be taken regarding issues of the generalisability of association findings, in order to avoid their premature use in, for instance predictive testing, in the face of this widespread heterogeneity (Cooper *et al.* 2008).

Understanding how aetiological factors act at a population level will be a critical step for the clinical application of new genomic knowledge to improve health outcomes (Ohlstein *et al.* 2000, Chanda and Caldwell, 2003, Goldstein *et al.* 2003b). Genetic knowledge will become clinically useful only when it is placed back in an epidemiological and public health context (Khoury *et al.* 2003, Burke, 2003, Merikangas and Risch, 2003, Kelada *et al.* 2003, Shostak, 2003). Very large, longitudinal, well characterised population-based studies drawn from multiple ethnic groups will be vital to the implementation of SNP-based gene discovery and in diagnostic tests for complex phenotypes in the outbred, highly admixed populations that increasingly characterise human societies today (Goldstein *et al.* 2003a) (see Chapter Six).

Rare alleles

Current attention in population-based association studies is focused almost entirely on genetic markers and aetiological variants that are common (>5% frequency). This is true for SNP detection studies, public SNP databases, the HapMap project and haplotype tagging approaches. Most sample collections are powered to detect only effects arising from common variants. There are several reasons for the common allele emphasis. The most often-cited relates to the 'common disease, common variant' hypothesis, which holds that the genetic influences on diseases of high population prevalence are old and are thus typically common. There are arguments and evidence for and against this hypothesis, as well as empirical support and counterexamples (Wright and Hastie, 2001, Hirschhorn *et al.* 2001, Terwilliger and Weiss, 2003, Bodmer and Bonilla, 2008, Mayo, 2007, Iyengar and Elston, 2007).

Another reason for the emphasis on common alleles is purely practical. Common diseases are assumed to be influenced by many genetic and environmental factors, all with a modest effect on the trait. If the genetic influences are rare, the sample sizes required to detect the modest effects become exceedingly large, rapidly reaching impossible levels (Risch, 2000, Zondervan and Cardon, 2004) (Figure 4.3). Thus, in the absence of 'low-hanging fruit' – genes with major effects on complex phenotypes – it is impractical to search for rare genetic effects using the allelic association design. This practical consideration supports the design of studies for only common alleles, under the expectation that many real effects will go undetected. This feature also explains why there appears to be little, if any, overlap between results being derived from the genome-wide assessment of SNP data and those derived from more classical family-based linkage scans for most diseases. Genome-wide linkage scans are well powered for the detection of rare variants with large effects that show patterns of inheritance within ascertained families. Data from the WTCCC GWAS (WTCCC, 2007) showed little evidence, as would be expected, for overlap with linkage studies (M.N. Weedon, E. Zeggini and M.I. McCarthy, personal communication), which is mainly due to the differing attributes of such analyses (Figure 4.4). However, this does not diminish the potential importance of the analysis of rare genetic variation. It is considered by many researchers that the presence of such variation may indeed go some way towards explaining the 'predictive gap' (also known as 'missing heritability') that exists between the apparently low levels of phenotypic variance already explained by common SNPs and the relatively high levels of heritability observed in family-based studies of the same outcomes (Bogardus, 2009, Maher, 2008).

Figure 4.4: Lack of overlap between loci for height defined by family-based linkage (grey numbered regions) and those defined by GWAS (grey dots)

Data from Perola *et al.* (2007) and Weedon *et al.* (2008). Figure courtesy of M. Weedon. The linkage and association study results shown were last updated in June 2007.

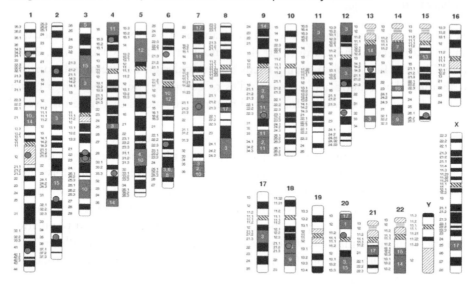

Allelic heterogeneity accentuates the problem of rare alleles. With the breast and ovarian cancer loci *BRCA1* and *BRCA2*, the phenotype results from a very large number of different mutations in the same gene(s) (Couch and Weber, 1996), so that many people have extremely rare or unique ('private') mutations. These rare mutations are unlikely to be detected by population-based association, no matter how large the sample size or the number of common SNPs genotyped (note that the *BRCA1* and *BRCA2* loci were identified by family-based linkage (Hall *et al.* 1990, Wooster *et al.* 1994)). Thus, there are genetic aetiologics that are simply not amenable to discovery by population association analysis (Weiss and Terwilliger, 2000, Terwilliger and Weiss, 2003). As these are not known a priori, it is important to emphasise that the vast SNP datasets being constructed, the HapMap project, enhanced genotyping capacity, and all the other resources being brought to bear on this problem will not always lead to gene discovery. It may be that selectively recalling and ascertaining the genotypes of family members of those participants who do not possess copies of common, validated risk alleles may be necessary to identify rare alleles.

As noted earlier, The 1000 Genomes Project will sequence 1,000 human genomes (Siva, 2008) over the next few years in order to provide much higher resolution data than the initial HapMap project. These data, some of which are already publicly available (The 1000 Genomes Project), will be particularly useful for investigating rarer alleles (down to 1% frequency in most populations).

Replication

Several recent articles have addressed the features of a 'good' genetic association study (Zondervan and Cardon, 2004, Chanock *et al.* 2007, Clarke *et al.* 2007) (see Chapter Five). This growing focus on study design has stemmed from the realisation that genetic association studies of complex phenotypes often either fail to discover susceptibility loci or fail to replicate studies that have discovered it (Ioannidis *et al.* 2001a, Lohmueller *et al.* 2003, Tabor *et al.* 2002, Weiss and Terwilliger, 2000, Goldstein *et al.* 2003a, Cardon and Bell, 2001, Terwilliger and Goring, 2000, Colhoun *et al.*, 2003). Despite the widespread use of genetic case-control studies, their inconsistency is a generally recognised limitation (Terwilliger and Goring, 2000, Weiss and Terwilliger, 2000). This lack of reproducibility is often ascribed to small samples with inadequate statistical power, biological and phenotypic complexity, population-specific LD, effect-size bias and population stratification (Ioannidis *et al.* 2001b, Goring *et al.* 2001, Weiss and Terwilliger, 2000, Risch, 2000). Other reasons for the non-replication of true positive association results include inter-investigator and inter-population heterogeneity in study design, analytical method, phenotype definition, genetic structure, environmental exposures and the markers genotyped. It is now routinely argued that large sample sizes (generally, thousands or tens of thousands), rigorous *p*-value thresholds and replication in multiple independent datasets are necessary for reliable results (Chanock *et al.* 2007). For many complex human diseases, the reality of multiple disease-predisposing genes of modest individual effect, gene-gene interactions, gene-environment interactions, heterogeneity of both genetic and environmental determinants of disease and low statistical power mean that both initial detection and replication of many genes will probably remain difficult.

A practical extension of the use of meta-analyses and the drive to discover replicable, albeit small, effects within association study frameworks has seen a move to the common use of multiple studies within GWAS publications and the formation of large, often phenotype-directed, consortia. A good example of the former is that of Zeggini and colleagues, who identified T2D risk loci and confirmed them through effective replication across the WTCCC, Finland-United States Investigation of NIDDM Genetics (FUSION) and Diabetes Genetics Initiative (DGI) studies (Zeggini *et al.* 2007). The simultaneous analysis of these three datasets alongside a large set of independent T2D cases and controls (provided by the Dundee T2D cohort) allowed the immediate replication and consolidation of top signals. This effort led to the identification of small but replicable association signals, and also yielded latent information as to the nature of these results. In the example of the fat mass and obesity related locus *FTO* it was observed that, in strata matched for body mass index, no association with T2D was present. This ultimately led to the investigation of *FTO* as an adipose-specific locus, but at the time was noted as an important source of informative heterogeneity.

A second, and important, demonstration of the ability of large consortia to detect relatively small but reliable genetic contributions to traits of interest comes from the genome-wide investigation of anthropometric measures (GIANT) consortium and its analysis of height and body mass index (Weedon *et al.* 2008, Weedon *et al.* 2007). In the case of body mass index, following the initial finding of the *FTO* gene (Frayling *et al.* 2007), the GIANT consortium has allowed the further discovery of loci with diminishingly small effects – the reliability of which have been guaranteed only by the analysis of over 80,000 individuals (Willer *et al.* 2009). Although the fraction of variance explained in these traits again confirms the 'predictive gap' left behind by association studies of this nature, these data provide a valuable perspective on the genetic architecture and aetiology of common phenotypic variation.

Ironically, the same advances in SNP genotyping and LD mapping that offer promise for association studies also highlight some of the difficulties that large SNP studies face. Decreasing costs mean that more SNPs will be genotyped and thus more spurious results will be obtained. This places a greater burden on establishing robustness by replication. However, many different definitions of replication are emerging. Descriptions of so-called 'confirmatory replication' are often attached to findings that appear non-confirmatory. For example, (1) different genetic markers are significantly associated in the follow-up study than those found in the original report; or (2) the same genetic markers show evidence for association in both studies, but with opposite alleles (that is, the 'disease' allele in the original report is the 'protective' allele in the follow-up); or (3) different phenotypes are reported to be associated in the initial and follow-up studies. Simulation studies have suggested that most such examples of 'allele flipping' are likely to be type 1 errors (Clarke *et al.* 2007).

The problem with these definitions of apparent confirmatory replication is that although they could reflect genuine replications because there are genetic reasons for their occurrence, they might also indicate false positives. The distinction between true replication and false positive is even more difficult to discern when samples from different populations are examined in the initial and follow-up studies. For the three examples given earlier in this paragraph, allelic heterogeneity could explain the first scenario, different population backgrounds the second (as apparent in animal models of disease (Mackay, 2001, Andersson and Georges, 2004)), and the third is consistent with genetic pleiotropy, in which one gene influences many phenotypes. These competing explanations point to the need for standardised definitions of replication, because some of the genetic explanations (such as the second) look biologically less plausible and compelling than other replication scenarios. Although there is no disputing the importance of heterogeneity within and between samples and genes, there is a risk that heterogeneity could be abused to frame negative follow-up studies in positive terms (Colhoun *et al.* 2003). In recognition of these issues, there is an increasing concern with rigorous standards for replication from journal editors and the research community (Chanock *et al.* 2007).

In general, studies showing similar results in terms of phenotypes tested and specific SNP associations may offer strong evidence for association; however, those that do not reveal such clear overlap – even those with positive association evidence – may require validation using other strategies or datasets. The current wave of consortia conducting pooled and meta-analyses of GWAS data (such as GIANT), cohorts for heart disease and ageing research in genomic epidemiology (CHARGE) and meta-analyses of glucose and insulin-related traits consortium (MAGIC) studies) need to approach these issues carefully lest replication lose its status as a gold standard for genetic association.

The future

Where does LD mapping stand today? For most complex human diseases, the reality of multiple disease-predisposing genes of modest individual effect, gene-gene interactions, gene-environment interactions, inter-population heterogeneity of both genetic and environmental determinants of disease and the concomitant low statistical power mean that both initial detection and replication of important genes will probably remain difficult, although not impossible. However, in addition to an improved understanding of the complexity of the task at hand, we also have some important new tools and a growing knowledge base that offer considerable prospects for the future success of gene discovery efforts. The technology for detecting SNPs has undergone rapid development, and increasingly complete catalogues of SNPs across the human genome have been constructed. A large number of groups are currently active in addressing methodological problems in LD mapping and haplotype approaches. Our growing understanding of the architecture of the human genome and the extent of human genetic variability – aided by projects such as International HapMap Project and the 1000 Genomes Project (Lang, 2008) – will probably accelerate our ability to use the tools at hand to map genes for many common conditions. However, almost all of the GWASs undertaken to date have made use of cases and controls almost exclusively from populations of European ancestry, and little is known about the frequency of risk alleles in other populations.

We stand at the threshold of the availability of several very large cohort opportunities throughout the world (see Chapter Six). These and other developments, taken together with a growing number of successful gene localisations for complex phenotypes, suggest that cautious optimism about our potential to discover the genes underlying common human diseases is justified. Another cause for hope has been the assimilation of genetic epidemiology into mainstream epidemiology and public health in many academic institutions. The growing engagement of epidemiologists in genetic research should ameliorate some of the difficulties that have plagued complex disease genetics, many of which can be blamed on poor study design and the over-interpretation of marginal results. Our understanding of complex disease pathophysiology has already begun to enter into the realm of clinical genetics (Mallal *et al.* 2008), and we have every reason to anticipate that the impact of genomics on clinical practice and on our understanding of biology and epidemiology will continue to accelerate. The work of human genome epidemiology and association analyses for the coming decade will centre around not only further discovery, but also the characterisation of validated genes across the lifecourse, the development of clinically useful risk models, and other translational projects (Palmer, 2004, Lindgren and McCarthy, 2008).

Acknowledgements

This work was supported in part by the Wind-over-Water Foundation (L.J. Palmer) and by a Wellcome Trust Principal Research Fellowship and NIH grant EY-12562 (L.R. Cardon).

References

Abecasis GR, Cherney SS, Cookson WOC, *et al.*, MERLIN: Multipoint engine for rapid likelihood inference. *American Journal of Human Genetics*, 2000; 67, 327.

Anderson CA, Pettersson FH, Barrett JC, *et al.*, Evaluating the effects of imputation on the power, coverage, and cost efficiency of genome-wide SNP platforms. *American Journal of Human Genetics*, 2008; 83, 112-9.

Andersson L, and Georges M, Domestic-animal genomics: deciphering the genetics of complex traits. *Nature Reviews Genetics*, 2004; 5, 202-12.

Angius A, Hyland FC, Persico I, *et al.*, Patterns of linkage disequilibrium between SNPs in a Sardinian population isolate and the selection of markers for association studies. *Human Heredity*, 2008; 65, 9-22.

Attia J, Ioannidis JP, Thakkinstian A, *et al.*, How to use an article about genetic association: A: Background concepts. *JAMA*, 2009; 301, 74-81.

Bacanu SA, Devlin B, and Roeder K, Association studies for quantitative traits in structured populations. *Genetic Epidemiology*, 2002; 22, 78-93.

Balding DJ, A tutorial on statistical methods for population association studies. *Nature Reviews Genetics*, 2006; 7, 781-91.

Barbujani G, Magagni A, Minch E, *et al.*, An apportionment of human DNA diversity. *Proceedings of the National Academy of Sciences USA*, 1997; 94, 4516-9.

Barrett JC, and Cardon LR, Evaluating coverage of genome-wide association studies. *Nature Genetics*, 2006; 38, 659-62.

Bodmer W, and Bonilla C, Common and rare variants in multifactorial susceptibility to common diseases. *Nature Genetics*, 2008; 40, 695-701.

Bogardus C, Missing heritability and GWAS utility. *Obesity (Silver Spring)*, 2009; 17, 209-10.

Botstein D, and Risch N, Discovering genotypes underlying human phenotypes: past successes for mendelian disease, future approaches for complex disease. *Nature Genetics*, 2003; 33 Suppl, 228-37.

Brookes AJ, The essence of SNPs. *Gene*, 1999; 8, 177-186.

Browning SR, Missing data imputation and haplotype phase inference for genome-wide association studies. *Human Genetics*, 2008; 124, 439-50.

Burke W, Genomics as a probe for disease biology. *New England Journal of Medicine*, 2003; 349, 969-74.

Burton PR, Clayton DG, Cardon LR, *et al.*, Association scan of 14,500 nonsynonymous SNPs in four diseases identifies autoimmunity variants. *Nature Genetics*, 2007; 39, 1329-37.

Burton PR, Hansell AL, Fortier I, *et al.*, Size matters: just how big is BIG?: Quantifying realistic sample size requirements for human genome epidemiology. *International Journal of Epidemiology*, 2008; 38, 1, 263-273.

Cardon LR, and Abecasis GR, Using haplotype blocks to map human complex trait loci. *Trends in Genetics*, 2003; 19, 135-40.

Cardon LR, and Bell JI, Association study designs for complex diseases. *Nature Reviews Genetics*, 2001; 2, 91-9.

Cardon LR, and Palmer LJ, Population stratification and spurious allelic association. *Lancet*, 2003; 361, 598-604.

Cardon LR, and Watkins H, Waiting for the working draft from the human genome project: A huge achievement, but not of immediate medical use. *British Medical Journal*, 2000; 320, 1221-1222.

Carlson CS, Eberle MA, Rieder MJ, *et al.*, Additional SNPs and linkage-disequilibrium analyses are necessary for whole-genome association studies in humans. *Nature Genetics*, 2003; 33, 518-21.

Carlson CS, Eberle MA, Rieder MJ, *et al.*, Selecting a maximally informative set of single-nucleotide polymorphisms for association analyses using linkage disequilibrium. *American Journal of Human Genetics*, 2004; 74, 106-20.

Cavalli-Sforza LL, Menozzi P, and Piazza A, *History and geography of human genes.* Princeton: Princeton University Press, 1994.

Chakravarti A, It's raining SNPs, hallelujah? [news]. *Nature Genetics*, 1998; 19, 216-7.

Chanda SK, and Caldwell JS, Fulfilling the promise: drug discovery in the post-genomic era. *Drug Discovery Today*, 2003; 8, 168-74.

Chanock SJ, Manolio T, Boehnke M, *et al.*, Replicating genotype-phenotype associations. *Nature*, 2007; 447, 655-60.

Chen L, Page GP, Mehta T, *et al.*, Single nucleotide polymorphisms affect both cis- and trans-eQTLs. *Genomics*, 2009; 93, 6, 501-508.

Chen Y, Zhu J, Lum PY, *et al.*, Variations in DNA elucidate molecular networks that cause disease. *Nature*, 2008; 452, 429-35.

Clarke GM, Carter KW, Palmer LJ, *et al.*, Fine Mapping versus Replication in Whole-Genome Association Studies. *American Journal of Human Genetics*, 2007; 81, 995-1005.

Colhoun HM, McKeigue PM, and Davey Smith G, Problems of reporting genetic associations with complex outcomes. *Lancet*, 2003; 361, 865-72.

Collins A, Lonjou C, and Morton NE, Genetic epidemiology of single-nucleotide polymorphisms. *Proceeding National Academy of Sciences USA*, 1999; 96, 15173-7.

Collins FS, Guyer MS, and Charkravarti A, Variations on a theme: cataloging human DNA sequence variation. *Science*, 1997; 278, 1580-1.

Collins FS, Patrinos A, Jordan E, *et al.*, New goals for the U.S. Human Genome Project: 1998-2003. *Science*, 1998; 282, 682-9.

Conrad DF, Jakobsson M, Coop G, *et al.*, A worldwide survey of haplotype variation and linkage disequilibrium in the human genome. *Nature Genetics*, 2006; 38, 1251-60.

Cooper RS, Tayo B, and Zhu X, Genome-wide association studies: implications for multiethnic samples. *Human Molecular Genetics*, 2008; 17, R151-5.

Couch FJ, and Weber BL, Mutations and polymorphisms in the familial early-onset breast cancer (BRCA1) gene. Breast Cancer Information Core. *Human Mutation*, 1996; 8, 8-18.

Crawford D C, Carlson CS, Rieder MJ, *et al.*, Haplotype Diversity across 100 Candidate Genes for Inflammation, Lipid Metabolism, and Blood Pressure Regulation in Two Populations. *American Journal of Human Genetics*, 2004; 74, 610-22.

Daly MJ, Rioux JD, Schaffner SF, *et al.*, High-resolution haplotype structure in the human genome. *Nature Genetics*, 2001; 29, 229-232.

Davey Smith G, Ebrahim S, Lewis S, *et al.*, Genetic epidemiology and public health: hope, hype, and future prospects. *Lancet*, 2005; 366, 1484-98.

Davey Smith G, Lawlor DA, Harbord R, *et al.*, Clustered environments and randomized genes: a fundamental distinction between conventional and genetic epidemiology. *PLoS Medicine*, 2007; 4, e352.

Davis RL, and Khoury MJ, A public health approach to pharmacogenomics and gene-based diagnostic tests. *Pharmacogenomics*, 2006; 7, 331-7.

Dawson E, Abecasis GR, Bumpstead S, *et al.*, A first generation linkage disequilibrium map of human chromosome 22. *Nature*, 2002; 418, 544-548.

De Bakker PI, Graham RR, Altshuler D, *et al.*, Transferability of tag SNPs to capture common genetic variation in DNA repair genes across multiple populations. *Pacific Symposium on Biocomputing*, 2006; 11, 478-86.

Devlin B, Roeder K, and Bacanu SA, Unbiased methods for population-based association studies. *Genetic Epidemiology*, 2001a; 21, 273-84.

Devlin B, Roeder K, and Wasserman L, Genomic control, a new approach to genetic-based association studies. *Theoretical Population Biology*, 2001b; 60, 155-66.

Durrant C, Zondervan KT, Cardon LR, *et al.*, Linkage disequilibrium mapping via cladistic analysis of single-nucleotide polymorphism haplotypes. *American Journal of Human Genetics*, 2004; 75, 35-43.

Ebrahim S, and Davey Smith G, Mendelian randomization: can genetic epidemiology help redress the failures of observational epidemiology? *Human Genetics*, 2008; 123, 15-33.

Edwards BJ, Haynes C, Levenstien MA, *et al.*, Power and sample size calculations in the presence of phenotype errors for case/control genetic association studies. *BMC Genetics*, 2005; 6, 18.

Edwards J, and Bartlett JM, Mutation and polymorphism detection: a technical overview. *Methods in Molecular Biology*, 2003; 226, 287-94.

Evans DM, Barrett JC, and Cardon LR, To what extent do scans of non-synonymous SNPs complement denser genome-wide association studies? *European Journal of Human Genetics*, 2008; 16, 718-23.

Evans DM, Marchini J, Morris AP, *et al.*, Two-stage two-locus models in genome-wide association. *PLoS Genetics*, 2006; 2, e157.

Ewens W, and Spielman R, The transmission/disequilibrium test: history, subdivision, and admixture. *American Journal of Human Genetics*, 1995; 57, 455-464.

Excoffier L, and Slatkin M, Maximum-likelihood estimation of molecular haplotype frequencies in a diploid population. *Molecular Biology and Evolution*, 1995; 12, 921-7.

Farber CR, van Nas A, Ghazalpour A, *et al.*, An Integrative Genetics Approach to Identify Candidate Genes Regulating Bone Density: Combining Linkage, Gene Expression and Association. *The Journal of Bone and Mineral Research*, 2008; 24, 1, 105-116.

Feinendegen L, Hahnfeldt P, Schadt EE, *et al.*, Systems biology and its potential role in radiobiology. *Radiation and Environmental Biophysics*, 2008; 47, 5-23.

Feldman MW, Lewontin RC, and King MC, Race: a genetic melting-pot. *Nature*, 2003; 424, 374.

Frayling TM, Timpson NJ, Weedon MN, *et al.*, A common variant in the FTO gene is associated with body mass index and predisposes to childhood and adult obesity. *Science*, 2007; 316, 889-94.

Frazer KA, Ballinger DG, Cox DR, *et al.*, A second generation human haplotype map of over 3.1 million SNPs. *Nature*, 2007; 449, 851-61.

Freedman ML, Reich D, Penney KL, *et al.*, Assessing the impact of population stratification on genetic association studies. *Nature Genetics*, 2004; 36, 388-393.

Gabriel S B, Schaffner SF, Nguyen H, *et al.*, The structure of haplotype blocks in the human genome. *Science*, 2002; 296, 2225-9.

Gauderman W, and Morrison J, (2006) *QUANTO 1.1: A computer program for power and sample size calculations for genetic-epidemiology studies*, http://hydra.usc.edu/gxe

Gibbs RA, Belmont JW, Hardenbol P, *et al.*, The International HapMap Project. *Nature*, 2003; 426, 789-96.

Golding, J, Pembrey M, and Jones R, ALSPAC – the Avon Longitudinal Study of Parents and Children. I. Study methodology. *Paediatric and Perinatal Epidemiology*, 2001; 15, 74-87.

Goldstein DB, Ahmadi KR, Weale ME, *et al.*, Genome scans and candidate gene approaches in the study of common diseases and variable drug responses. *Trends in Genetics*, 2003a; 19, 615-22.

Goldstein DB, Tate SK and Sisodiya SM, Pharmacogenetics goes genomic. *Nature Reviews Genetics*, 2003b; 4, 937-47.

Gonzalez CA, The European Prospective Investigation into Cancer and Nutrition (EPIC). *Public Health Nutrition*, 2006; 9, 124-6.

Goring HH, Terwilliger JD, and Blangero J, Large upward bias in estimation of locus-specific effects from genomewide scans. *American Journal of Human Genetics*, 2001; 69, 1357-69.

Gray IC, Campbell DA, and Spurr NK, Single nucleotide polymorphisms as tools in human genetics. *Human Molecular Genetics*, 2000; 9, 2403-8.

Gu CC, Yu K, Ketkar S, *et al.*, On transferability of genome-wide tagSNPs. *Genetic Epidemiology*, 2008; 32, 89-97.

Hahn LW, Ritchie MD, and Moore JH, Multifactor dimensionality reduction software for detecting gene-gene and gene-environment interactions. *Bioinformatics*, 2003; 19, 376-82.

Hall JM, Lee MK, Newman B, *et al.*, Linkage of early-onset familial breast cancer to chromosome 17q21. *Science*, 1990; 250, 1684-9.

Hirschhorn JN, Lindgren CM, Daly MJ, *et al.*, Genomewide linkage analysis of stature in multiple populations reveals several regions with evidence of linkage to adult height. *American Journal of Human Genetics*, 2001; 69, 106-16.

Hoggart CJ, Clark TG, De Iorio M, *et al.*, Genome-wide significance for dense SNP and resequencing data. *Genetic Epidemiology*, 2008a; 32, 179-85.

Hoggart CJ, Whittaker JC, De Iorio M, *et al.*, Simultaneous analysis of all SNPs in genome-wide and re-sequencing association studies. *PLoS Genetics*, 2008b; 4, e1000130.

Hu C, Jia W, Zhang W, *et al.*, An evaluation of the performance of HapMap SNP data in a Shanghai Chinese population: analyses of allele frequency, linkage disequilibrium pattern and tagging SNPs transferability on chromosome 1q21-q25. *BMC Genetics*, 2008; 9, 19.

Huang RC, Burke V, Newnham JP, *et al.*, Perinatal and childhood origins of cardiovascular disease. *International Journal of Obesity (Lond)*, 2006; 31, 236–244.

Hunter DJ, Gene-environment interactions in human diseases. *Nature Reviews Genetics*, 2005; 6, 287-98.

Ioannidis JP, Gwinn M, Little J, *et al.*, A road map for efficient and reliable human genome epidemiology. *Nature Genetics*, 2006; 38, 3-5.

Ioannidis JP, Ntzani EE, Trikalinos TA, *et al.*, Replication validity of genetic association studies. *Nature Genetics*, 2001a; 29, 306-9.

Ioannidis JP, Ntzani EE, Trikalinos TA, *et al.*, Replication validity of genetic association studies. *Nature Genetics*, 2001b; 29, 306-309.

Iyengar SK, and Elston RC, The genetic basis of complex traits: rare variants or "common gene, common disease"? *Methods in Molecular Biology*, 2007; 376, 71-84.

Janssens AC, and van Duijn CM, Genome-based prediction of common diseases: methodological considerations for future research. *Genome Medicine*, 2009; 1, 20.

Jaquish CE, The Framingham Heart Study, on its way to becoming the gold standard for Cardiovascular Genetic Epidemiology? *BMC Medical Genetics*, 2007; 8, 63.

Johnson GC, Esposito L, Barratt BJ, *et al.*, Haplotype tagging for the identification of common disease genes. *Nature Genetics*, 2001; 29, 233-237.

Jorde LB, Linkage disequilibrium and the search for complex disease genes. *Genome Research*, 2000; 10, 1435-44.

Jorde LB, Watkins WS, Carlson M, *et al.*, Linkage disequilibrium predicts physical distance in the adenomatous polyposis coli region. *American Journal of Human Genetics*, 1994; 54, 884-98.

Kanehisa M, and Bork P, Bioinformatics in the post-sequence era. *Nature Genetics*, 2003; 33 Suppl, 305-10.

Ke X, Hunt S, Tapper W, *et al.*, The impact of SNP density on fine-scale patterns of linkage disequilibrium. *Human Molecular Genetics*, 2004; 13, 577–588.

Kelada SN, Eaton DL, Wang SS, *et al.*, The role of genetic polymorphisms in environmental health. *Environmental Health Perspectives*, 2003; 111, 1055-64.

Keller MP, Choi Y, Wang P, *et al.*, A gene expression network model of type 2 diabetes links cell cycle regulation in islets with diabetes susceptibility. *Genome Research*, 2008; 18, 706-16.

Khoury MJ, McCabe LL, and McCabe ER, Population screening in the age of genomic medicine. *New England Journal of Medicine*, 2003; 348, 50-8.

Khoury MJ, and Wacholder S, Invited commentary: from genome-wide association studies to gene-environment-wide interaction studies--challenges and opportunities. *American Journal of Epidemiology*, 2009; 169, 227-30; discussion 234-5.

Kruglyak L, The use of a genetic map of biallelic markers in linkage studies. *Nature Genetics*, 1997; 17, 21-4.

Kruglyak L, The road to genome-wide association studies. *Nature Reviews Genetics*, 2008; 9, 314-8.

Kruglyak L, and Nickerson DA, Variation is the spice of life. *Nature Genetics*, 2001; 27, 234-6.

Kuhner MK, Beerli P, Yamato J, *et al.*, Usefulness of single nucleotide polymorphism data for estimating population parameters. *Genetics*, 2000; 156, 439-47.

Lander E, and Kruglyak L, Genetic dissection of complex traits: guidelines for interpreting and reporting linkage results. *Nature Genetics*, 1995; 11, 241-247.

Lang L, Three sequencing companies join the 1000 genomes project. *Gastroenterology*, 2008; 135, 336-7.

Lawrence R, Evans DM, Morris AP, *et al.*, Genetically indistinguishable SNPs and their influence on inferring the location of disease-associated variants. *Genome Research*, 2005; 15, 1503-10.

Li Q, and Yu K, Improved correction for population stratification in genome-wide association studies by identifying hidden population structures. *Genetic Epidemiology*, 2007; 32: 215–226.

Lindgren CM, and McCarthy MI, Mechanisms of disease: genetic insights into the etiology of type 2 diabetes and obesity. *National Clinical Practice Endocrinology and Metabolism*, 2008; 4, 156-63.

Little R, and Yau L, Intent-to-treat analysis for longitudinal studies with drop-outs. *Biometrics*, 1996; 52, 1324-33.

Liu N, Zhang K, and Zhao H, Haplotype-association analysis. *Advances in Genetics*, 2008; 60, 335-405.

Lohmueller KE, Pearce CL, Pike M, *et al.*, Meta-analysis of genetic association studies supports a contribution of common variants to susceptibility to common disease. *Nature Genetics*, 2003; 33, 177-82.

Loos RJ, Lindgren CM, Li S, *et al.*, Common variants near MC4R are associated with fat mass, weight and risk of obesity. *Nature Genetics*, 2008; 40, 768-75.

Mackay TF, The genetic architecture of quantitative traits. *Annual Review of Genetics*, 2001; 35, 303-39.

Maher B, Personal genomes: The case of the missing heritability. *Nature*, 2008; 456, 18-21.

Mallal S, Phillips E, Carosi G, *et al.*, HLA-B*5701 screening for hypersensitivity to abacavir. *New England Journal of Medicine*, 2008; 358, 568-79.

Mallinckrodt CH, Sanger TM, Dube S, *et al.*, Assessing and interpreting treatment effects in longitudinal clinical trials with missing data. *Biological Psychiatry*, 2003; 53, 754-60.

Manolio TA, Brooks LD, and Collins FS, A HapMap harvest of insights into the genetics of common disease. *The Journal of Clinical Investigation*, 2008; 118, 1590-605.

Marchini J, Cardon LR, Phillips MS, *et al.*, The effects of human population structure on large genetic association studies. *Nature Genetics*, 2004a; 36, 512-7.

Marchini J, Cardon LR, Phillips MS, *et al.*, The effects of human population structure on large genetic association studies. *Nature Genetics*, 2004b; 36, 512–517.

Mayo O, The rise and fall of the common disease-common variant (CD-CV) hypothesis: how the sickle cell disease paradigm led us all astray (or did it?). *Twin Research and Human Genetics*, 2007; 10, 793-804.

McCarroll SA, Extending genome-wide association studies to copy-number variation. *Human Molecular Genetics*, 2008; 17, R135-42.

McKeigue PM, Mapping genes that underlie ethnic differences in disease risk: methods for detecting linkage in admixed populations, by conditioning on parental admixture. *American Journal of Human Genetics*, 1998; 63, 241-51.

Merikangas KR., and Risch N, Genomic priorities and public health. *Science*, 2003; 302, 599-601.

Mira MT, Alcais A, Nguyen VT, *et al.*, Susceptibility to leprosy is associated with PARK2 and PACRG. *Nature*, 2004; 427, 636-40.

Molenberghs G, Williams PL, and Lipsitz SR, Prediction of survival and opportunistic infections in HIV-infected patients: a comparison of imputation methods of incomplete CD4 counts. *Statistics in Medicine*, 2002; 21, 1387-408.

Moskvina V, and Schmidt KM, On multiple-testing correction in genome-wide association studies. *Genetic Epidemiology*, 2008; 32, 567-73.

Mote VL, and Anderson RL, An Investigation of the Effect of Misclassification on the Properties of Chi-2-Tests in the Analysis of Categorical Data. *Biometrika*, 1965; 52, 95-109.

Myles S, Davison D, Barrett J, *et al.*, Worldwide population differentiation at disease-associated SNPs. *BMC Medical Genomics*, 2008; 1, 22.

Nebert DW, Zhang G, and Vesell ES, From human genetics and genomics to pharmacogenetics and pharmacogenomics: past lessons, future directions. *Drug Metabolism Review*, 2008; 40, 187-224.

Ness AR, The Avon Longitudinal Study of Parents and Children (ALSPAC)--a resource for the study of the environmental determinants of childhood obesity. *European Journal of Endocrinology*, 2004; 151 Suppl 3, U141-9.

Nickerson DA, Whitehurst C, Boysen C, *et al.*, Identification of clusters of biallelic polymorphic sequence-tagged sites (pSTSs) that generate highly informative and automatable markers for genetic linkage mapping. *Genomics*, 1992; 12, 377-87.

Niu T, Qin ZS, Xu X, *et al.*, Bayesian haplotype inference for multiple linked single-nucleotide polymorphisms. *American Journal of Human Genetics*, 2002; 70, 157-69.

Ohlstein EH, Ruffolo RR Jr, and Elliott JD, Drug discovery in the next millennium. *Annual Review of Pharmacology and Toxicology*, 2000; 40, 177-91.

Orr N, and Chanock S, Common genetic variation and human disease. *Advances in Genetics*, 2008; 62, 1-32.

Overall AD and Nichols RA, A method for distinguishing consanguinity and population substructure using multilocus genotype data. *Molecular Biology and Evolution*, 2001; 18, 2048-56.

Palmer LJ, The New Epidemiology: putting the pieces together in complex disease aetiology. *International Journal of Epidemiology*, 2004; 33, 925-8.

Palmer LJ, (2007) UK Biobank: bank on it. *Lancet*, 369, 1980-2.

Palmer LJ, and Cardon LR, Shaking the tree: mapping complex disease genes with linkage disequilibrium. *Lancet*, 2005; 366, 1223-34.

Palmer LJ, and Cookson WOCM, Genomic approaches to understanding asthma. *Genome Research*, 2000; 10, 1280-1287.

Palmer LJ, and Cookson WOCM, Using Single Nucleotide Polymorphisms (SNPs) as a means to understanding the pathophysiology of asthma. *Respiratory Research*, 2001; 2, 102-112.

Patil N, Berno A J, Hinds DA, *et al.*, Blocks of limited haplotype diversity revealed by high-resolution scanning of human chromosome 21. *Science*, 2001; 294, 1719-23.

Peltonen L, and McKusick VA, Genomics and medicine. Dissecting human disease in the postgenomic era. *Science*, 2001; 291, 1224-9.

Perola M, Sammalisto S, Hiekkalinna T, *et al.*, Combined genome scans for body stature in 6,602 European twins: evidence for common Caucasian loci. *PLoS Genetics*, 2007; 3, e97.

Phillips MS, Lawrence R, Sachidanandam R, *et al.*, Chromosome-wide distribution of haplotype blocks and the role of recombination hot spots. *Nature Genetics*, 2003; 33, 382-7.

Price AL, Patterson NJ, Plenge RM, *et al.*, Principal components analysis corrects for stratification in genome-wide association studies. *Nature Genetics*, 2006; 38, 904-9.

Pritchard JK, and Rosenberg NA, Use of unlinked genetic markers to detect population stratification in association studies. *American Journal of Human Genetics*, 1999; 65, 220-8.

Pritchard JK, Stephens M, Rosenberg NA, *et al.*, (2000) Association mapping in structured populations. *American Journal of Human Genetics*, 2000; 67, 170-81.

Raghunathan TE, What do we do with missing data? Some options for analysis of incomplete data. *Annual Review of Public Health*, 2004; 25, 99-117.

Reich DE, Gabriel SB, and Altshuler D, Quality and completeness of SNP databases. *Nature Genetics*, 2003; 33, 457-8.

Rice TK, Schork NJ, and Rao DC, Methods for handling multiple testing. *Advances in Genetics*, 2008; 60, 293-308.

Risch N, Burchard E, Ziv E *et al.*, Categorization of humans in biomedical research: genes, race and disease. *Genome Biology*, 2002; 3, 2007.

Risch N, and Merikangas K, The future of genetic studies of complex human diseases. *Science*, 1996; 273, 1516-1517.

Risch NJ, Searching for genetic determinants in the new millennium. *Nature*, 2000; 405, 847-56.

Ritchie MD, Hahn LW, Roodi N, *et al.*, Multifactor-dimensionality reduction reveals high-order interactions among estrogen-metabolism genes in sporadic breast cancer. *American Journal of Human Genetics*, 2001; 69, 138-47.

Rosenberg NA, Li LM, Ward R, *et al.*, Informativeness of genetic markers for inference of ancestry. *American Journal of Human Genetics*, 2003; 73, 1402-22.

Rosner B, *Fundamental of biostatistics.* Boston: PWS-Kent, 1990.

Saccone NL, Saccone SF, Goate AM, *et al.*, In search of causal variants: refining disease association signals using cross-population contrasts. *BMC Genetics*, 2008; 9, 58.

Sachidanandam R, Weissman D, Schmidt SC, *et al.*, A map of human genome sequence variation containing 1.42 million single nucleotide polymorphisms. *Nature*, 2001; 409, 928-933.

Salari K, Choudhry S, Tang H, *et al.*, Genetic admixture and asthma-related phenotypes in Mexican American and Puerto Rican asthmatics. *Genetic Epidemiology*, 2005; 29, 76-86.

Satten GA, Flanders WD, and Yang Q, Accounting for unmeasured population substructure in case-control studies of genetic association using a novel latent-class model. *American Journal of Human Genetics*, 2001; 68, 466-77.

Saxena R, Voight BF, Lyssenko V, *et al.*, Genome-wide association analysis identifies loci for type 2 diabetes and triglyceride levels. *Science*, 2007; 316, 1331-6.

Schadt EE, Novel integrative genomics strategies to identify genes for complex traits. *Animal Genetics*, 2006; 37 Suppl 1, 18-23.

Schadt EE, Molony C, Chudin E, *et al.*, Mapping the genetic architecture of gene expression in human liver. *PLoS Biology*, 2008; 6, e107.

Schaid DJ, Relative efficiency of ambiguous vs. directly measured haplotype frequencies. *Genetic Epidemiology*, 2002; 23, 426-43.

Schaid DJ, Rowland CM, Tines DE, *et al.*, Score tests for association between traits and haplotypes when linkage phase is ambiguous. *American Journal of Human Genetics*, 2002; 70, 425-34.

Schork NJ, Fallin D, and Lanchbury JS, Single nucleotide polymorphisms and the future of genetic epidemiology. *Clinical Genetics*, 2000; 58, 250-64.

Schulze TG, Zhang K, Chen YS, *et al.*, Defining haplotype blocks and tag single-nucleotide polymorphisms in the human genome. *Human Molecular Genetics*, 2004; 13, 335-42.

Scuteri A, Sanna S, Chen WM, *et al.*, Genome-Wide Association Scan Shows Genetic Variants in the FTO Gene Are Associated with Obesity-Related Traits. *PLoS Genetics*, 2007; 3, e115.

Sham PC, Rijsdijk FV, Knight J, *et al.*, Haplotype association analysis of discrete and continuous traits using mixture of regression models. *Behavior Genetics*, 2004; 34, 207-14.

Shifman S, Kuypers J, Kokoris M, *et al.*, Linkage disequilibrium patterns of the human genome across populations. *Human Molecular Genetics*, 2003; 12, 771-6.

Shostak S, Locating gene-environment interaction: at the intersections of genetics and public health. *Social Science and Medicine*, 2003; 56, 2327-42.

Shriver MD, Smith MW, Jin L, *et al.*, Ethnic-affiliation estimation by use of population-specific DNA markers. *American Journal of Human Genetics*, 1997; 60, 957-64.

Sieberts SK, and Schadt EE, Moving toward a system genetics view of disease. *Mammalian Genome*, 2007; 18, 389-401.

Siva N, 1000 Genomes project. *Nature Biotechnology*, 2008; 26, 256.

Slatkin M, Linkage disequilibrium--understanding the evolutionary past and mapping the medical future. *Nature Reviews Genetics*, 2008; 9, 477-85.

Stafford N, Scientists meet to agree framework for European biobank. *British Medical Journal*, 2008; 336, 467.

Stallings RL, Ford AF, Nelson D, *et al.*, Evolution and distribution of (GT)n repetitive sequences in mammalian genomes. *Genomics*, 1991; 10, 807-15.

Steemers FJ, and Gunderson KL, Whole genome genotyping technologies on the BeadArray platform. *Biotechnology Journal*, 2007; 2, 41-9.

Stephens M, Smith NJ, and Donnelly P, A new statistical method for haplotype reconstruction from population data. *American Journal of Human Genetics*, 2001; 68, 978-89.

Tabor HK, Risch NJ, and Myers RM, Opinion: Candidate-gene approaches for studying complex genetic traits: practical considerations. *Nature Reviews Genetics*, 2002; 3, 391-7.

Tachmazidou I, Verzilli CJ, and De Iorio M, Genetic association mapping via evolution-based clustering of haplotypes. *PLoS Genetics*, 2007; 3, e111.

Templeton AR, Cladistic approaches to identifying determinants of variability in multifactorial phenotypes and the evolutionary significance of variation in the human genome. *Ciba Found Symp*, 1996; 197, 259-77.

Terwilliger JD, and Goring HH, Gene mapping in the 20th and 21st centuries: statistical methods, data analysis, and experimental design. *Human Biology*, 2000; 72, 63-132.

Terwilliger JD, and Weiss KM, Confounding, ascertainment bias, and the blind quest for a genetic 'fountain of youth'. *Annals of Medicine*, 2003; 35, 532-44.

The 1000 Genomes Project, www.1000genomes.org/page.php

The International HapMap Project, The International HapMap Project. *Nature*, 2003; 426, 789-96.

The International HapMap Project, A haplotype map of the human genome. *Nature*, 2005; 437, 1299-320.

Thomas S, Porteous D, and Visscher PM, Power of direct vs. indirect haplotyping in association studies. *Genetic Epidemiology*, 2004; 26, 116-24.

Toivonen HT, Onkamo P, Vasko K, et al., Data mining applied to linkage disequilibrium mapping. *American Journal of Human Genetics*, 2000; 67, 133-45.

Varmus H, Genomic empowerment: the importance of public databases. *Nature Genetics*, 2003; 35 Suppl 1, 3.

Verbeke G, and Molenberghs G, *Linear mixed models for longitudinal data*. New York: Springer, 2000.

von Bubnoff A, Next-generation sequencing: the race is on. *Cell*, 2008; 132, 721-3.

Wang DG, Fan JB, Siao CJ, et al., Large-scale identification, mapping, and genotyping of single- nucleotide polymorphisms in the human genome. *Science*, 1998; 280, 1077-82.

Watkins WS, Zenger R, O'Brien E, et al., Linkage disequilibrium patterns vary with chromosomal location: a case study from the von Willebrand factor region. *American Journal of Human Genetics*, 1994; 55, 348-55.

Weedon MN, Lango H, Lindgren CM, et al., Genome-wide association analysis identifies 20 loci that influence adult height. *Nature Genetics*, 2008; 40, 575-83.

Weedon MN, Lettre G, Freathy RM, et al., A common variant of HMGA2 is associated with adult and childhood height in the general population. *Nature Genetics*, 2007; 39, 1245-50.

Weiss KM, and Terwilliger JD, How many diseases does it take to map a gene with SNPs? *Nature Genetics*, 2000; 26, 151-7.

White IR, Moodie E, Thompson SG, et al., A modelling strategy for the analysis of clinical trials with partly missing longitudinal data. *International Journal of Methods in Psychiatric Research*, 2003; 12, 139-50.

Willer CJ, Speliotes EK, Loos RJ, et al., Six new loci associated with body mass index highlight a neuronal influence on body weight regulation. *Nature Genetics*, 2009; 41, 25-34.

Wolfe KH, and Li WH, Molecular evolution meets the genomics revolution. *Nature Genetics*, 2003; 33 Suppl, 255-65.

Wooster R, Neuhausen SL, Mangion J, *et al.*, Localization of a breast cancer susceptibility gene, BRCA2, to chromosome 13q12-13. *Science*, 1994; 265, 2088-90.

Wright AF, and Hastie ND, (2001) Complex genetic diseases: controversy over the Croesus code. *Genome Biology*, 2001; 2, comment 2007.

WTCCC, Genome-wide association study of 14,000 cases of seven common diseases and 3,000 shared controls. *Nature*, 2007; 447, 661-78.

Xing J, Witherspoon DJ, Watkins WS, *et al.*, HapMap tagSNP transferability in multiple populations: general guidelines. *Genomics*, 2008; 92, 41-51.

Yamada R, Primer: SNP-associated studies and what they can teach us. *Nature Clinical Practice Rheumatology*, 2008; 4, 210-7.

Yang JO, Hwang S, Oh J, *et al.*, An integrated database-pipeline system for studying single nucleotide polymorphisms and diseases. *BMC Bioinformatics*, 2008; 9, Suppl 12, S19.

Yeager M, Xiao N, Hayes RB, *et al.*, Comprehensive resequence analysis of a 136 kb region of human chromosome 8q24 associated with prostate and colon cancers. *Human Genetics*, 2008; 124, 161-70.

Zavattari P, Deidda E, Whalen M, *et al.*, Major factors influencing linkage disequilibrium by analysis of different chromosome regions in distinct populations: demography, chromosome recombination frequency and selection. *Human Molecular Genetics*, 2000; 9, 2947-2957.

Zeggini E, Weedon MN, Lindgren CM, *et al.*, Replication of genome-wide association signals in UK samples reveals risk loci for type 2 diabetes. *Science*, 2007; 316, 1336-41.

Zerhouni E, Medicine. The NIH Roadmap. *Science*, 2003; 302, 63-72.

Zhang W, Ratain MJ, and Dolan ME, The HapMap Resource is Providing New Insights into Ourselves and its Application to Pharmacogenomics. *Bioinformatics and Biology Insights*, 2008; 2, 15-23.

Zheng G, and Tian X, The impact of diagnostic error on testing genetic association in case-control studies. *Statistical Medicine*, 2005; 24, 869-82.

Zheng J, Moorhead M, Weng L, *et al.*, High-throughput, high-accuracy array-based resequencing. *Proceedings of the National Academy of Sciences USA*, 2009; 106, 6712-7.

Zheng SL, Sun J, Wiklund F, *et al.*, Cumulative association of five genetic variants with prostate cancer. *New England Journal of Medicine*, 2008; 358, 910-9.

Zhu J, Wiener MC, Zhang C, *et al.*, Increasing the power to detect causal associations by combining genotypic and expression data in segregating populations. *PLoS Computational Biology*, 2007; 3, e69.

Zhu J, Zhang B, and Schadt EE, A systems biology approach to drug discovery. *Advances in Genetics*, 2008; 60, 603-35.

Ziegler A, Konig IR, and Thompson JR, Biostatistical aspects of genome-wide association studies. *Biom J*, 2008; 50, 8-28.

Zondervan KT, and Cardon LR, The complex interplay among factors that influence allelic association. *Nature Reviews Genetics*, 2004; 5, 89-100.

FIVE

A question of standards: what makes a good genetic association study?

Andrew T. Hattersley, Mark I. McCarthy

Summary

Genetic association studies are central to efforts to identify and characterise genomic variants underlying susceptibility to multi-factorial disease. However, a major source of frustration has been the difficulty of obtaining robust replication of initial association findings. Much of this inconsistency can be attributed to inadequacies in study design, implementation and interpretation, with the use of inadequately powered sample groups a paramount concern. Several additional factors have an impact on the quality of any given association study – an appropriate sample recruitment strategy, logical variant selection, minimal genotyping error, relevant data analysis and valid interpretation are all essential contributors to the generation of robust findings. Replication has a vital role in demonstrating that associations observed reflect interesting biological processes rather than methodological quirks. An unbiased view of the evidence for and against any particular association needs to focus on study quality, rather than the headline significance value. This chapter discusses these and related issues predominantly as it relates to candidate genes studies rather than genome–wide association studies.

Introduction

Optimal study design for the detection and characterisation of genes contributing to the development of common multi-factorial traits has been a subject of considerable and growing interest over the previous decade. Much of the recent focus has been on association study designs. Although theoretical analyses have often emphasised the power of association methodology (Risch and Merikangas, 1996), only limited novel insights had arisen from candidate gene studies (Lohmueller *et al.* 2003) before the advent of genome-wide association studies (GWASs) (Wellcome Trust Case Control Consortium, 2007; see also Chapters One, Three and Four). A major source of historical frustration and confusion has been the frequency with which initial positive findings are not confirmed in subsequent studies (Ioannidis *et al.* 2001; Hirschhorn *et al.* 2002; Ioannidis *et al.* 2003; Lohmueller *et al.* 2003; Chanock *et al.* 2007; Clarke *et al.* 2007). Replication remains an area of critical concern, both for candidate gene studies and GWASs (Chanock *et al.* 2007).

Part of the explanation for such inconsistency of replication may lie in biological factors. There may be genuine differences between studies in terms of the frequency of a particular susceptibility variant, genetic background or relevant environmental exposures that affect the capacity to obtain replication. However, many of these apparently contradictory results can be attributed to questions of study design, implementation and interpretation (Cardon and Palmer, 2003; Daly *et al.* 2005; de Bakker *et al.* 2005; Altshuler *et al.* 2007; Clarke *et al.* 2007; Zondervan and Cardon, 2007). Concentrating on practical issues related to these matters, this chapter aims to allow the reader who lacks an in-depth knowledge of genetic epidemiology to assess the quality of association studies, and to better appreciate the inferences that can legitimately be made. It will also contribute to ongoing discussions on the development of standards for association studies, designed both to raise the overall quality of studies performed and to facilitate robust meta-analysis (Little *et al.* 2002; Ioannidis *et al.* 2006; Khoury *et al.* 2007) Although GWASs represent the current cutting edge of genetic epidemiological research on complex diseases, candidate gene studies retain a key role in investigations of the aetiology of such diseases. This chapter focuses on candidate gene studies; genome-wide association scans are discussed in Chapter Four.

The objective of performing an association study

The objective of any association study is deceptively simple – to determine whether a statistical relationship exists between genomic variation at one or more sites and phenotypic variation. Phenotypic variation is usually represented by the presence/absence of a disease or by levels of a disease-related trait (see Chapter Three). The archetypal case–control study design compares two groups that have been ascertained specifically because they are expected to differ appreciably in their prevalence of disease-susceptibility alleles. Provided the sampling has been appropriate (ensuring that cases and controls have similar ethnic background, for example) (Cardon and Palmer 2003), the detection of a significant difference in variant frequency between the two groups (a significant association) is consistent with the hypothesis that either the variant typed influences trait susceptibility or that a second variant, in linkage disequilibrium with the first, does so.

Key to grappling with the limitations of much of the existing literature reporting association data for multi-factorial traits is the need to appreciate the small effect sizes that are to be expected. The modest extent of familial clustering of many complex traits, and the failure, with notable exceptions, to detect large susceptibility effects through linkage studies (Altmuller *et al.* 2001), clearly indicate that the number of large genetic effects for any given disease is likely to vary from zero to 'a few'. Evidence from the few variants consistently shown to be associated with common disease endorses this view. In general, the susceptibility variants identified to date are either common, but have only modest relative risk – for example, *PPARG* and type 2 diabetes (Altshuler *et al.* 2000); or uncommon with substantial relative risks – for example, factor V Leiden and thrombosis (Bertina *et al.* 1994). In either case, detection by association is not straightforward (Risch and Merikangas, 1996). Except for HLA effects on autoimmune disease, there are few confirmed associations due to a common variant (>10% allele frequency) with a relative risk exceeding 2.0. Examples include those between variation in *APOE* and Alzheimer's disease (Corder *et al.* 1993) and between variation in the gene encoding complement factor H and age–related macular degeneration (Edwards, 2005; Hageman *et al.* 2005; Haines *et al.* 2005; Klein *et al.* 2005; Zareparsi *et al.* 2005) (Table 5.1).

Many association studies performed to date have had only limited power to detect true susceptibility effects on this scale, and even less power to exclude a gene from involvement in a disease or trait of interest. Changing this is not only desirable, but with collaborative efforts to collect much larger sample sets, improved genotyping and analytical technologies and recent advances in bioinformatics, this is now possible. It requires that more attention be paid to critical appraisal of study design, implementation and interpretation, and a better understanding of the parameters that define a 'good' association study. In the remainder of this chapter, the main issues that need to be addressed when evaluating such research will be described.

Choosing a good candidate gene

There are around 20,000 genes in the human genome, and it is unlikely that more than a few hundred of these make a meaningful contribution to variation in any single phenotype. As a consequence, the prior probability that any gene selected at random will truly influence a given trait is extremely low. Evidence from a range of sources (Table 5.2) can be used to identify genes (candidates) with higher prior odds for phenotypic involvement: the overwhelming majority of association studies have featured genes selected using one or more of these criteria. Prior information of this kind should also inform the interpretation of association findings: it seems reasonable to demand a higher level of statistical evidence for genes with very little supporting biological information before interest is provoked, or significance attributed (Risch and Merikangas, 1996; Colhoun *et al.* 2003; Wacholder *et al.* 2004; Chanock *et al.* 2007).

However, it is also important to realise that evaluating candidacy is a notoriously imprecise art. Poor understanding of the molecular mechanisms underlying most complex traits (itself one of the main justifications for gene discovery efforts) means that precise quantification of the prior odds associated with any given gene is rarely feasible. Many of the methods listed in Table 5.2 do a rather inadequate job of picking out true susceptibility genes, especially if deployed in isolation (McCarthy *et al.* 2003). It is also worth noting that detection of a true association requires not only that the gene product be involved in pathways relevant to the development of the trait of interest, but also that the gene contains variants capable of influencing its regulation or function.

Table 5.1: Examples of some (non-MHC) polymorphisms or haplotypes that have shown consistent association with complex disease

Disease	Gene	Polymorphism	Approximate frequency of the disease-associated allele	Approximate odds ratio for disease-associated allele	References
Thrombophilia	*F5*	Leiden Arg506Gln	0.03	4	Bertina *et al.* 1994
Crohn's disease	*CARD15*	3 SNPs	0.06 (composite)	4.6	Hugot *et al.* 2001
Alzheimer's disease	*APOE*	ε2/3/4	0.15	3.3	Corder *et al.* 1993; Rubinsztein and Easton 1999
Type 1 diabetes	*PTPN22*	Arg620Trp	0.16	1.6	Smyth *et al.* 2004, Bottini *et al.* 2004
Osteoporotic fractures	*COL1A1*	Sp1 restriction site	0.19	1.3	Mann and Ralston, 2003, Mann *et al.* 2001
Prostate cancer	*EST AW183883*	DG8S737	0.19 (Europeans)	1.6	Amundadottir *et al.* 2006
Age-related macular degeneration	*HF1/CFH*	Tyr402His (and others)	0.30	2.5	Zareparsi *et al.* 2005, Hageman *et al.* 2005, Haines *et al.* 2005, Klein *et al.* 2005, Edwards *et al.* 2005
Type 2 diabetes	*TCF7L2*	Rs7903146	0.30	1.5	Grant *et al.* 2006, Groves *et al.* 2006
Type 2 diabetes	*KCNJ11*	Glu23Lys	0.36	1.23	Gloyn *et al.* 2003
Type 1 diabetes	*CTLA4*	Thr17Ala	0.36	1.27	Ueda *et al.* 2003, Marron *et al.* 1997
Graves' disease	*CTLA4*	Thr17Ala	0.36	1.6	Chistiakov and Turakulov, 2003
Coeliac disease	*MYO9B*	Rs2305764	0.38	1.6	Monsuur *et al.* 2005
Type 1 diabetes	*INS*	5 VNTR	0.67	1.2	Bennett and Todd, 1996
Bladder cancer	*GSTM1*	Null (gene deletion)	0.70	1.28	Engel *et al.* 2002
Type 2 diabetes	*PPARG*	Pro12Ala	0.85	1.23	Altshuler *et al.* 2000

The table includes only those polymorphisms or haplotypes identified in the era before genome-wide association studies. Examples are shown in increasing order of the frequency of the disease-associated allele.

Table 5.2: Criteria for selection of candidate genes

	Explanation	Advantages	Disadvantages	Examples
Biology	Known or presumed function of the protein encoded implicated in known or presumed biology of the disease or trait	Good when pathophysiology known, eg autoimmune disease or thrombophilia	Not as good when primary pathophysiology unknown, eg hypertension or type 2 diabetes	Factor V Leiden in thrombophilia (Bertina et al. 1994)
Pharmacology	Gene encodes a protein implicated (eg as target) in mechanism of action of disease- or trait-modifying drug	Evidence that modification of pathway by small molecules can influence trait, suggests that genetic variation may do likewise	Treatment may not act on the aetiological pathway	PPARG in type 2 diabetes (Altshuler et al. 2000)
Animal models	Identification of genes influencing related traits in animal models offers candidates for testing in humans	Provides clear functional links between gene dysfunction and whole body phenotype	Species differences may exist both in physiology and in patterns of genetic variation	ApoAV and hypertriglyceridaemia (Pennacchio et al. 2001)
Monogenic or syndromic forms of the disease	Genes in which rare mutations lead to monogenic or syndromal forms of disease may also show common genetic variation that predisposes to polygenic disease	Rare monogenic disorders establish the gene has a critical function and indicates lack of compensation or plasticity	An appropriate monogenic disease may not exist	Monogenic diabetes and type 2 diabetes (reviewed in McCarthy, 2004)
Positional information	Genome-wide scans for linkage or association may indicate regions with a high probability of containing a susceptibility gene	Genes that account for reproducible linkage peaks in genome scans are likely to represent major susceptibility genes	Regions of interest defined by linkage remain large. Linkage studies are usually underpowered and will not detect all susceptibility genes	APOE and Alzheimer's disease (Corder et al. 1993)
Prior association data	Previous studies showing association with a gene or a meta-analysis of previous studies indicate that variation in the gene is likely to have an aetiological role	Previous positive studies can give some of the strongest prior knowledge for examining a gene	Caution is needed: initial association studies generally overestimate the effect size of the variant tested	PPARG, KCNJ11, CAPN10 in type 2 diabetes (Altshuler et al. 2000; Gloyn et al. 2003; Weedon et al. 2003)

Selection of genetic variants

To guarantee detection of all possible disease-associated variants at a given gene, one would need to examine, in sufficiently large sample sets, *every* base at which variation could conceivably alter gene function or expression. Only then can one be confident that an association has not been missed simply because the wrong markers have been typed (Zondervan and Cardon, 2004). At present, this counsel of perfection remains unrealistic: with current genotyping technologies, it is simply too expensive to examine several hundreds of variants in several thousands of subjects for every gene of legitimate interest. Given that exhaustive typing is impractical, choices must be made, and the strategy used to define the subset of variants to be typed has a substantial impact on the power and quality of the study. In recent years, greater understanding of the nature and extent of human genomic variation has enabled more logical strategies for variant selection. Nevertheless, it is important to appreciate that variant selection always represents a pragmatic compromise.

There are two complementary approaches to the selection of variants. The 'tagging' approach seeks to exploit the extensive linkage disequilibrium seen in many parts of the genome. By typing the subset of variants that captures a disproportionate amount of the information in common regional haplotypes, it may be possible to maintain power while making considerable savings in genotyping (Johnson *et al.* 2001). In its most conservative form, tagging simply avoids redundant typing of sets of variants that are in complete linkage disequilibrium with each other, but a variety of approaches that allow more sophisticated tag selection have emerged in recent years (Carlson *et al.* 2004a, 2004b; Stram, 2004; de Bakker *et al.* 2005) (see also Chapter Four). Advocates of the 'common disease, common variant' hypothesis argue, on a variety of theoretical (Reich and Lander, 2001) and empirical (Lohmueller *et al.* 2003) grounds, that many of the alleles influencing susceptibility to common complex traits will themselves be common. If so, then the typing of regional tag SNPs, selected specifically to capture such common genomic variation, should provide an efficient approach for detecting complex trait susceptibility alleles (Gabriel *et al.* 2002; Zondervan and Cardon, 2004). This view has gained considerable support with recent successes from genome-wide association scans (Wellcome Trust Case Control Consortium, 2007; Frayling *et al.* 2007; Samani, 2007; see also Chapter Four). However, the capacity of common tags to capture rare variants is poor (Zeggini *et al.* 2005). Evidence that such rare variants can make a substantial contribution to variation in disease-related phenotypes emphasises that the tagging approach will have its limits, at least for some traits (Cohen *et al.* 2005).

The second approach to variant selection aims to incorporate assessments of the likely functional impact of variation within a gene or region of interest. Those variants thought most likely to influence gene expression or function (irrespective of their relationship to local haplotype structure) (Tabor *et al.* 2002) are then prioritised for typing. Unfortunately, predicting the functional credentials of most variants remains extremely difficult. Non-synonymous coding variants are obvious targets, but assessment of the potential regulatory impact of intronic variants or those lying several kilobases upstream of a gene remains poor (Hudson, 2003). One critical issue is the need to define the extent of the regulatory elements influencing a given gene. Reports of association between haplotypes surrounding the recently discovered beta-cell promoter of the *HNF4A* gene and type 2 diabetes demonstrate the difficulties (Silander *et al.* 2004; Love-Gregory *et al.* 2004). This promoter, which lies 46 kb upstream of the coding region, was only identified a decade after the delineation of the coding sequence (Thomas *et al.* 2001; Boj *et al.* 2001). Increasingly, application of cross-species sequence comparisons to identify conserved non-coding sequences likely to represent regulatory elements (Loots *et al.* 2002) and high-throughput experimental tools for defining sites of gene regulation (Knight *et al.* 2003) promise to aid both variant selection and the interpretation of association studies.

Until such methods are established, much weight will be placed on the detailed functional assessment of those variants that have shown some preliminary evidence for association – the rationale being that demonstration of a functional effect provides biological corroboration, enhancing the probability that the statistical association is genuine. Although reasonable, considerable caution is required in interpreting such findings. Firstly, *in vitro* functional studies have intrinsic limitations: it can be hard to know how to interpret results that suggest that the functional effects of a given variant are only observed in certain cell lines, under certain experimental conditions, by particular investigators. Secondly, it is evident that allelic variation in gene expression is commonplace and may be present in most genes (Lo *et al.* 2003). Thus, evidence that a particular variant influences the expression of a gene may add little to a questionable association finding, especially in the absence of any evidence that differential expression of the gene in question can be causally related to the development of the trait of interest.

Appropriateness of typed samples

Appropriate subject selection is central to the design of any association study. In classical epidemiology, the prospective cohort study design is often considered the gold standard. Although cohort studies can provide an understanding of risk at the population level, and therefore remain an essential weapon in the armoury of genetic epidemiologists, they are typically rather inefficient tools for the initial stages of gene discovery. Unless the disease is very common, the study samples they generate will be highly unbalanced (that is, they will have far fewer individuals with disease than without), and the nested case-control samples that emerge are often relatively modest in size. In addition, the unselected nature of the cases may compromise power, especially when compared with samples deliberately enriched for genetic aetiology and disease homogeneity. A study of the widely replicated association between variation in the *TCF7L2* gene and type 2 diabetes (Grant *et al.* 2006) demonstrated significantly lower relative risks among unselected cases, as compared with cases ascertained for positive family history and early onset

(Groves *et al.* 2006). Given these limitations, the case-control study remains the workhorse of genetic association studies, and the most pertinent issues relate to the ascertainment of the two subject groups.

In many ways, collection of cases is the easier task, given that clinical presentation facilitates recruitment. However, investigators have to make several crucial decisions, explicitly or implicitly, that can influence the outcome of any given study. One relates to subject characterisation: is it better to have a larger number of cases, albeit less well characterised, accepting that some misclassification and heterogeneity is inevitable, or to strive for phenotypic homogeneity, albeit at the cost of reduced sample size? Unfortunately, no generic answer is possible – the 'correct' strategy depends on disease- and study-specific factors, which are both known (for example, the cost and specificity of the phenotyping tools used) and unknown (the genetic architecture of the condition). A more profitable focus may lie in the selection of cases likely to be enriched for genetic susceptibility. Even without straying over the boundary from multi-factorial into monogenic disease, there are good reasons to expect selection on the basis of strong family history (Teng and Risch, 1999) and/or early age of onset (Frayling *et al.* 2003) to increase the susceptibility allele frequency difference between cases and controls, and for given sample size, to improve power. When searching for associations within regions known to be linked to the disease of interest, a further boost to the allele frequency difference can be obtained by selecting on the family-specific evidence for linkage and/or by using allele-sharing information to select those subjects showing maximal sharing with other affected relatives (Fingerlin *et al.* 2004). However, it is essential to remember that, although careful selection of cases (and controls, see below) should provide a valid test of association but with improved power, reliable estimation of population-based parameters (relative risk, population-attributable risk) is not possible using extreme samples and will require analysis of population-based cohorts.

Therefore, although there is no universally correct recipe for case ascertainment, the decisions taken by investigators in this regard may have a significant impact on the power of their studies in often unpredictable ways. This fact may help to explain some inconsistencies in outcome between studies.

Issues related to control selection have been extensively discussed (Colhoun *et al.* 2003; Cardon and Palmer, 2003; Zondervan and Cardon, 2004). It is, of course, essential that the controls are selected from the same population as the cases, or that approaches (such as genomic control or direct estimation of admixture with ancestry-informative markers) are used to correct for any latent population stratification (Bacanu *et al.* 2000). The question of whether or not to select controls on the basis of phenotype and/or age remains a major issue of debate.

Compared with population controls (that is, a sample considered representative of the population from which the cases were ascertained), the use of 'hypernormal' controls (for example, older subjects known to be free of the disease of interest, or in the case of prostate cancer, men with low prostate-specific antigen levels [Eeles *et al.* 2008]) would be expected to improve power by increasing the difference in susceptibility allele frequency between cases and controls. However, this benefit is generally not substantial (Colhoun *et al.* 2003), and can easily be outweighed by the costs associated with defining a hypernormal population (the need to phenotype subjects for disease status, the potential for inadvertent selection for other phenotypes such as survivor effects). One increasingly favoured option is the use of large control cohorts of clear provenance, often nationally representative (Wellcome Trust Case Control Consortium, 2007). One such example is the UK MRC 1958 Birth Cohort, composed of individuals born in a single week during March 1958, who have undergone extensive longitudinal follow-up (Power and Elliott, 2006). Such population cohorts can potentially provide controls for studies in a wide range of diseases (as in the Wellcome Trust Case Control Consortium: www.wtccc.org.uk)[1], although when the mean age of cases differs appreciably from that of the control cohort, survivor bias becomes a concern. There are considerable benefits associated with building up a large body of genotype, phenotype and quality control data on a single control cohort. The value of family-based association resources as an alternative source of controls is discussed later in this chapter.

Study size

The key determinant of quality in an association study is sample size (Ioannidis *et al.* 2003). With limited numbers of common genes with large effects on offer, studies must be powered to detect variants that are either common (but have low relative risk) or rarer (but with higher relative risk). As Table 5.3 demonstrates, this effectively means sample sizes in the thousands (Campbell *et al.* 1995). Rare variants with low relative risks are largely beyond the reach of genetic epidemiology because of the massive sample size that would be needed. It is important to note that these calculations assume that the susceptibility variant itself (or a marker with which it is in complete linkage disequilibrium) has been typed, which is

Table 5.3: Approximate sample sizes required to detect significant association given differing effect sizes and allele frequencies for the predisposing allele

γ (Allelic odds ratio)	Susceptibility allele frequency in controls					
	1%	5%	10%	20%	30%	40%
1.1	221,927	46,434	24,626	13,987	10,759	9,505
1.2	58,177	12,217	6,509	3,730	2,896	2,581
1.3	25,055	5,702	3,051	1,763	1,380	1,240
1.5	10,604	2,249	1,213	712	566	516
2.0	3,193	687	377	229	188	177
4.0	598	134	78	52	46	47

Power = 90%, two-sided α = 0.001. Calculations assume a multiplicative effect on disease risk (the homozygous susceptibility genotype has a penetrance that exceeds that of the heterozygote by a factor γ, the genotype relative risk, and that of the wild type homozygote by γ^2). Under such a model, each allele has independent effects on disease risk, and the allelic odds ratio is also equal to γ. The sample sizes presented are the total number of cases required in a case-control study in which controls are present in equal numbers. These sample size derivations assume the best case scenario in which the susceptibility variant itself (or a perfect proxy) has been typed.

very much a best case scenario. The apparent success of much smaller studies than those implied by Table 5.3 in identifying interesting associations might suggest that these sample size calculations are overly pessimistic. However, small initial studies only infrequently produce the correct result (Ioannidis *et al.* 2003; Wacholder *et al.* 2004) and, even when they do, are notably likely to overestimate the true effect size (Lohmueller *et al.* 2003).

What are the practical implications of these sobering power calculations? In truth, it is hard to make any case for performing even initial studies on small samples. Should such a study generate positive findings, the putative association needs to be replicated in a second, ideally larger, sample to provide a more realistic assessment of the reproducibility and size of the effect. Given that it is clear that the only way to obtain a robust estimate of modest susceptibility effects is through large studies (Altshuler *et al.* 2000), there is an increasing emphasis on national and international collaborations that allow appropriate large-scale replications to be undertaken at an early stage in the assessment of any given gene or region (Ioannidis *et al.* 2006; Khoury *et al.* 2007). Ideally, groups with access to multiple cohorts should type and report on all available samples when publishing positive results – as is increasingly happening (Frayling *et al.* 2007). However, large sample size alone is no guarantee of scientific validity. Increased sample size reduces the effects of sampling error but brings with it an increased danger of false positives, as hypothesis testing becomes exquisitely sensitive to the consequences of small bias effects due, for example, to population stratification (Marchini *et al.* 2004; Chanock *et al.* 2007).

Accuracy of genotyping

Most association studies are based on the implicit assumption that the genotypes obtained are completely accurate. However, even with the best technologies available, a proportion of assays will be unreliable; and the performance of earlier genotyping methods will be poorer still. Even well regarded genotyping laboratories using powerful new technologies assessed under optimal conditions report overall error rates close to 1% (and SNP-specific rates up to 3%) (Mein *et al.* 2000), so error rates of a few percent are not untypical (Bogardus *et al.* 1999).

Genotyping error can have a marked effect on the outcome of an association study. Most interest has focused on the extent to which random genotyping error reduces the power to detect true case-control differences (Gordon *et al.* 2002; Kang *et al.* 2004). For example, under typical assumptions, each 1% rise in genotyping error might require a sample size increase of 2-8% to maintain constant type 1 and type 2 error rates (Gordon *et al.* 2002). Random error rates of a few per cent therefore have an appreciable, though not calamitous, effect on power.

Of greater concern are situations in which systematic genotyping error generates a bias away from the null, leading to an increased danger of making a false attribution of association. Given the low prior probability of association expected of most variants, and the impact of publication and other biases that favour promulgation of positive findings (Ioannidis, 1998; Lohmueller *et al.* 2003), studies affected by genotyping error of this type are almost certainly disproportionately represented in the literature. Some study designs – such as family-based association tests using case-parent triads – are inherently prone to bias away from the null hypothesis, whether the errors are detected (and the relevant genotypes, individuals or families removed from analysis) or not (Curtis and Sham, 1995; Mitchell *et al.* 2003; Knapp and Becker, 2004). This somewhat counterintuitive consequence arises because only certain configurations of genotyping error generate Mendelian consistencies detectable within triads: the remaining undetected errors lead to apparent overtransmission of common alleles to affected offspring and to false-positive associations (Mitchell *et al.* 2003). In case–control studies, batch–related differences in genotyping performance can pose a particular problem. In many laboratories, it remains standard practice to store, and subsequently genotype, different sample sets (for example, cases and controls) on separate plates. As a result, any variation between batches in genotyping accuracy and/or tendency to preferentially reject particular genotypes (usually heterozygotes) will translate into between–group differences in genotype distribution. Given that even modest levels of genotyping error can have a serious impact on the accuracy of haplotypic reconstruction (Kirk and Cardon, 2002), the consequences of such errors can be profound. More seriously, recent data have demonstrated the potential for subtle differences in DNA quality between cases and controls to translate into systematic genotyping differences (such as non-random missing data), with consequent inflation of the type 1 error rate (Clayton *et al.* 2005).

Reducing the adverse impact of genotyping error on association studies requires advances in three areas. First, there is a transparent need for more accurate genotyping platforms. Methods with substantially improved performance (Fan *et al.* 2006) are becoming available, but, at the same time, the move towards genome-wide association magnifies the potential for mistakes. Second, genotyping errors need to be taken into greater consideration, with more widespread use of methods that establish and monitor the performance of each assay and reduce possible sources of error and bias (see Table 5.4). Even with the best platforms, a proportion of assays will continue to misbehave as a result of, for example, allelic dropout caused by variation within primer binding sites (Ewen *et al.* 2000). Third, information on genotyping performance needs to become an essential component of the metadata reported with any association study (Little *et al.* 2002), providing journals (and their reviewers and readers) with the information required for critical appraisal and facilitating future meta-analyses (which should incorporate some understanding of error estimates).

Table 5.4a: Detecting genotyping error in association studies

Method of detecting error	Question asked
Duplicate genotype assignment	What is the discordance rate between two operators 'scoring' the same genotypes?
Duplicate genotyping on same assay	What is the discrepancy rate when a proportion of samples (ideally 10-20%) are re-genotyped using the same method?
Duplicate genotyping on another assay	What is the discrepancy rate when a proportion of samples are re-genotyped using a different method?
Blank control wells	Is there any contamination of the PCR reagents? Is the plate oriented correctly?
Expected allele frequencies	Are allele (and/or haplotype) frequencies in line with those expected from previous data on other similar ethnic groups?
Hardy-Weinberg equilibrium	Are genotype frequencies consistent with Hardy-Weinberg equilibrium? (Note that modest departures, particularly in case samples, may be evidence of association)
Between-run consistency	When comparing results from different batches of the same assay, are there any 'outlier' batches with extreme allele and/or haplotype distributions that need to be targeted for repeat?
Mendelisation	Where related individuals have been typed, are genotypes consistent with Mendelian expectation? (Note that in simple family structures typed for biallelic markers only a minority of genotyping errors will generate Mendelian inconsistency)
Assay performance metrics	Where the particular genotyping method provides these, are 'quality scores' for individual genotypes and/or batches satisfactory?
Linkage disequilibrium relationships/haplotype structure	Where several adjacent SNPs have been typed in a region of limited linkage disequilibrium, do haplotype relationships suggest any fluctuations in genotyping performance? Appearance of haplotypes that have never previously been seen can be a very sensitive measure of error

Table 5.4b: Minimising genotyping error in association studies

Ways to minimise error	Details
Assay design	Robust assay design incorporating, where possible, quality checks (such as obligate restriction sites in a PCR- restriction fragment length polymorphism assay); confirm that assay detects all genotypes accurately by comparison with reference samples
Monitor assay quality on assay-specific basis	Derive and monitor quality control metrics (see part (a)) for each assay
Complete genotyping	Batch-related biases are most likely when genotyping call rates are low, so beware of any assay with poor call rate
Mix sample sets within batches	Ensure that cases and controls are mixed on the same plate (for example by intercalating 96-well plates onto a single 384-well plate)
If in doubt, retype	No single measure will detect all available errors and correcting all detectable errors will not reduce the error rate to zero. If the quality control metrics indicate assay failure, redesign the assay and retype

Appropriateness of the analysis

Each type of association study – case-control, family-based or within-cohort – raises a host of analytical issues that can act as traps for the unwary. Ready access to so many analytical programs can easily lead to inappropriate usage if the underlying assumptions are not clearly stated or appreciated. Consider, for instance, the question of haplotype reconstruction. There has been an explosion in methods for dealing with the important task of inferring haplotypes from unphased genotype data (as obtained in a sample of unrelated individuals) (Clark, 1990; Excoffier and Slatkin, 1995; Stephens *et al.* 2001; Niu *et al.* 2002; Stephens and Donnelly, 2003). However, the conceptual and computational differences between these methods translate into substantial differences in performance and, sometimes, in outcome (Niu *et al.* 2002; Stephens and Donnelly 2003). Similarly, when inferring haplotypes within pedigrees, substantial errors can arise with methods that inappropriately assume that the typed markers are in linkage equilibrium (Schaid *et al.* 2002).

Even those who are experienced in the field may find it almost impossible to establish whether appropriate methods have been used, and the extent to which the results obtained are robust. One recommendation is to urge researchers to make raw genotype data freely available (Page *et al.* 2003), though doing so raises confidentiality and consent issues. Sufficient genotype data may accrue on individuals in well typed and easily identified subsets (for example members of a population isolate, or recruits to a cohort defined by occupation or birth week) to render individual study participants potentially identifiable. The best guarantor of probity is likely to remain clear evidence of significant participation from recognised experts in statistical genetics during study design, data analysis and peer review. Additional reassurance comes from demonstration that the most important findings from a study have been robust to analysis using several complementary methods: a result that is dependent on a particular program or method is of dubious value.

Appropriateness of the interpretation

The perceived unreliability of association studies has generated much discussion regarding the level of evidence required before an association can be declared 'proven'. The emphasis has generally been on the need for greater stringency (Risch and Merikangas, 1996; Colhoun *et al.* 2003). On the basis that there are likely to be around 10^6 variants within the genome capable (in principle) of influencing any given human trait, Risch and Merikangas (1996) suggested that an appropriate threshold might be a *p*-value of 5×10^{-8} (that is, the standard 0.05 corrected for 10^6 tests). Colhoun *et al.* (2003), arguing from a Bayesian perspective, suggested that a threshold of 5×10^{-5} should be adequate to constrain the false discovery rate (that is, the proportion of associations declared positive that are, in fact, false). The issue of appropriate statistical thresholds for 'significance' and the closely related issue of appropriate corrections for multiple testing remain areas of very active interest (Benjamini and Yekutieli, 2005; de Bakker *et al.* 2005; Dudbridge *et al.* 2006; Clarke *et al.* 2007; Wellcome Trust Case Control Consortium, 2007; Hoggart *et al.* 2008; Rice *et al.* 2008)

As with the equivalent values for linkage studies (Lander and Kruglyak, 1995), such thresholds provide useful benchmarks for the interpretation of association findings, whether from a single study or a meta-analysis. However, a distinction needs to be made between thresholds and standards for assigning proof beyond reasonable doubt (which, given the history of association studies, should clearly tend towards the stringent), and those required for dissemination of association findings (which should require that the study has been well designed and performed). To limit publication to studies that conclusively 'prove' association (or, alternatively, those that achieve the difficult task of demonstrating conclusively that variation within a gene plays no role in disease susceptibility) would paralyse research, because few single studies would reach such levels of conviction. Although the proportionate increases in sample size required to satisfy more stringent criteria are surprisingly modest (Table 5.5), these still translate into substantial increases in absolute numbers beyond the scope of many current collections. Moreover, any policy insisting on such stringent criteria for publication would further complicate the task of obtaining an unbiased overview of all the data, positive or negative, available for a given association. Many good quality (largely negative) studies would not be disseminated, leaving the published research even more prone to bias.

Table 5.5: The effect of differing statistical significance levels on sample size

α-value	Susceptibility allele frequency in controls					
	1%	5%	10%	20%	30%	40%
0.05	13,599	2,866	1,533	886	694	623
0.01	19,258	4,058	2,171	1,255	982	883
0.001	27,055	5,702	3,051	1,763	1,380	1,240
5×10^{-5}	36,869	7,770	4,157	2,403	1,881	1,690
5×10^{-8}	58,678	12,369	6,617	3,825	2,994	2,690

Figures denote the sample size required to detect significant association (power = 90%) for different values of α (the threshold for declaring significance) assuming an allelic odds ratio of 1.3, given differing allele frequencies for the predisposing allele or haplotype. Assumptions are the same as those for Table 5.3.

The fundamental problem is that the headline *p*-value of an association study has very little to do with experimental quality. Well performed studies (featuring large, appropriate subject samples, robust low-error genotyping and clear primary hypotheses) will advance knowledge even if none of the association tests performed reaches significance at the chosen threshold. In contrast, relatively few associations first reported in small sample sizes prove reliable in larger datasets (Ioannidis *et al.* 2001; Ioannidis *et al.* 2003). Studies of the role of the *ACE* insertion/deletion variant in myocardial infarction (Keavney *et al.* 2000), and of the Pro12Ala SNP in *PPARG* in type 2 diabetes (Altshuler *et al.* 2000), illustrate this point. In the former, larger studies made it clear that the associations reported in small case-control samples had overestimated the true effect size, most likely as a result of publication bias (Keavney *et al.* 2000). In the latter, large studies have shown that many of the early case-control studies were simply too small to provide any useful estimate of the true effect size (Altshuler *et al.* 2000).

Of course, the logistical limitations of conventional modes of scientific dissemination mean that experimental quality cannot be the sole consideration for publication. Journals must take scientific interest of findings into account; and given that only a small proportion of variants are likely to show association to any given phenotype, it is legitimate to regard positive findings as having intrinsically greater impact. The solution to this quandary is a rigorous application of criteria to ensure study quality, combined with the development of acceptable alternative forums for the deposition and dissemination of all good quality association data. In the mean time, there is a need for the peer-review process to weigh study quality and the apparent biological interest of the headline findings more equitably (Chanock *et al.* 2007).

Another issue in relation to the interpretation of study results is the need for more complete statements of prior hypotheses and the range of analyses performed in a given study. All too often, in the effort to produce at least one *p*-value that reaches nominal significance, exploratory analyses arising from post hoc subdivision and stratification of the data are presented as major findings. One aspect of multiple testing is relatively easy to solve: it is straightforward to report the number of variants typed in a particular study (Redden and Allison, 2003) and to adjust for this using standard methods based on the Bonferroni correction or alternatives such as the false discovery rate (Storey and Tibshirani, 2003; Rice *et al.* 2008). These adjustments can readily take correlations between the typed markers caused by linkage disequilibrium into account (Nyholt, 2004) (Rice *et al.* 2008).

However, it is more difficult to allow for the proliferation of analyses that might be performed at each locus. For example, association may be sought at the level of the allele or the genotype: if the latter, several genetic models (dominant or recessive) can be tested (Schaid, 1996). If several markers have been typed, analyses of haplotype or diplotype frequency become possible (Epstein and Satten, 2003). Analyses may consider the effects of stratification by, or adjustment for, factors such as gender or disease subtype or age; additional phenotypes may be considered as outcome variables (for example age at disease onset, or another phenotype related to disease). Evidence of interaction effects (gene-gene or gene-environment) may be sought, whether or not main effects are evident (Kraft, 2004). Where case-parent triads are typed, it becomes possible to test for parent-of-origin and a variety of epigenetic effects (Weinberg, 1999). Of course, any of these analytical manoeuvres may be entirely justified in any given study, on the basis of prior biological hypotheses, or the desire to replicate specific findings arising from previous studies. However, where this is not the case, such repeated analyses will, if no correction is made, significantly inflate the overall type 1 error of the study.

In practice, the high degree of correlation between these analyses may make determination of the extent of any correction extremely difficult.

The challenge is to avoid making false attribution of associations based on post hoc analyses, without ruining the capacity to undertake potentially informative data exploration in what may be expensively acquired samples of richly characterised individuals. Part of the answer must be a clearer statement of prior hypotheses (including, potentially, some form of pre-study registration of intent), and a more complete description of all the different analyses undertaken. Most importantly, demonstrating that hypotheses generated from post hoc analyses in one sample can be confirmed in directed analyses in another provides an essential tool for establishing credibility.

Conclusions

Individual association studies can be viewed as stages on a journey that starts with ignorance and (hopefully) ends with a clear and robust assessment of whether or not variation at a given locus contributes to disease susceptibility. Only exceptionally will conclusive evidence be forthcoming from a single study. As Page *et al.* (2003) point out, the major purpose of replication in association studies is not only to improve the statistical significance of the findings. Replication studies also provide insurance from the errors and biases that may unavoidably afflict any individual study. They also amplify confidence that any associations uncovered reflect processes that are biologically interesting (that is, a variant that truly influences disease susceptibility), rather than methodological inadequacies (for example, inappropriate control groups, genotyping error, investigator biases or over-elaborate data exploration) (Lykken, 1968; Page *et al.* 2003; Maraganore *et al.* 2005; Palmer and Cardon, 2005; Goris *et al.* 2006).

Acknowledgements
We thank many colleagues in the genetics of type 2 diabetes and other polygenic disease for their useful discussion on these topics, particularly Steven Wiltshire, Eleftheria Zeggini and Chris Groves (Oxford), and Tim Frayling, Michael Weedon and Kirsten Ward (Exeter).

References
Altmuller J, Palmer LJ, Fischer G, *et al.*, Genomewide scans of complex human diseases: true linkage is hard to find. *American Journal of Human Genetics*, 2001; 69, 936–50.

Altshuler D, Daly M, Guilt beyond a reasonable doubt. *Nature Genetics*, 2007; 39, 7, 813–5.

Altshuler D, Hirschhorn JN, Klannemark M, *et al.*, The common PPARg Pro12Ala polymorphism is associated with decreased risk of type 2 diabetes. *Nature Genetics*, 2000; 26, 76–80.

Amundadottir LT, Sulem P, Gudmundsson J, *et al.*, A common variant associated with prostate cancer in European and African populations. *Nature Genetics*, 2006; 38, 652-658.

Bacanu SA, Devlin B, Roeder K, The power of genomic control. *American Journal of Human Genetics*, 2000; 66, 1933-44.

Barrett JC, Cardon LR, Evaluating coverage of genome-wide association studies. *Nature Genetics*, 2006; 38, 659-62.

Benjamini Y, Yekutieli D, Quantitative trait Loci analysis using the false discovery rate. *Genetics*, 2005; 171, 2, 783-90.

Bennett ST, Todd JA, Human type 1 diabetes and the insulin gene: principles of mapping polygenes. *Annual Review of Genetics*, 1996; 30, 343-70.

Bertina RM, Koeleman BP, Koster T, *et al.*, Mutation in blood coagulation factor V associated with resistance to activated protein C. *Nature*, 1994; 369, 64-7.

Bogardus ST Jr, Concato J, Feinstein AR, Clinical epidemiological quality in molecular genetic research: the need for methodological standards. *JAMA*, 1999; 281, 1919-26.

Boj SF, Parrizas M, Maestro MA, *et al.*, A transcription factor regulatory circuit in differentiated pancreatic cells. *Proceedings of the National Academy of Sciences USA*, 2001; 98, 14481-14486.

Bottini N, Musumeci L, Alonso A, *et al.*, A functional variant of lymphoid tyrosine phosphatase is associated with type I diabetes. *Nature Genetics*, 2004; 36, 337-338.

Campbell MJ, Julious SA, Altman DG, Estimating sample sizes for binary, ordered categorical, and continuous outcomes in two group comparisons. *British Medical Journal*, 1995; 311, 1145-1148.

Cardon LR, Palmer LJ, Population stratification and spurious allelic association. *Lancet*, 2003; 361, 598-604.

Carlson CS, Eberle MA, Rieder MJ, *et al.*, Selecting a maximally informative set of single-nucleotide polymorphisms for association analyses using linkage disequilibrium. *American Journal of Human Genetics*, 2004a; 74, 106-120

Carlson CS, Eberle MA, Kruglyak L, Nickerson DA, Mapping complex disease loci in whole-genome association studies. *Nature*, 2004b; 429, 446-452

Chanock SJ, Manolio T, Boehnke M, *et al.* Replicating genotype-phenotype associations. *Nature*, 2007; 447, 7145, 655-60.

Chistiakov DA, Turakulov RI, CTLA-4 and its role in autoimmune thyroid disease. *Journal of Molecular Endocrinology*, 2003; 31, 21-36.

Clark AG, Inference of haplotypes from PCR-amplified samples of diploid populations. *Molecular Biology and Evolution*, 1990; 7, 111-22.

Clarke GM, Carter KW, Palmer LJ, *et al.*, Fine Mapping versus Replication in Whole-Genome Association Studies. *American Journal of Human Genetics*, 2007; 81, 5, 995-1005.

Clayton DG, Walker NM, Smyth DJ, *et al.*, Population structure, differential bias and genomic control in a large-scale, case-control association study. *Nature Genetics*, 2005; 37, 1243-6

Cohen J, Pertsemlidis A, Kotowski IK, *et al.*, Low LDL cholesterol in individuals of African descent resulting from frequent nonsense mutations in PCSK9. *Nature Genetics*, 2005; 37, 161–5.

Colhoun HM, McKeigue PM, Davey Smith G, Problems of reporting genetic associations with complex outcomes. *Lancet*, 2003; 361,865–72

Corder EH, Saunders AM, Strittmatter WJ, *et al.*, Gene dose of apolipoprotein E type 4 allele and the risk of Alzheimer's disease in late onset families. *Science*, 1993; 261, 921–3.

Curtis D, Sham PC, A note on the application of the transmission disequilibrium test when a parent is missing. *American Journal of Human Genetics*, 1995; 56, 811–812.

Daly MJ, Altshuler D, Partners in crime. *Nature Genetics*, 2005; 37,4, 337–8.

de Bakker PI, Yelensky R, Pe'er I, *et al.*, Efficiency and power in genetic association studies. *Nature Genetics*, 2005; 37, 1217–23.

de Bakker PI, Yelensky R, Pe'er I, *et al.*, Efficiency and power in genetic association studies. *Nature Genetics*, 2005; 37, 11, 1217–23.

Dudbridge F, Gusnanto A, Koeleman BP, Detecting multiple associations in genome-wide studies. *Human Genomics*, 2006; 2, 5, 310–7.

Edwards AO, Ritter R 3rd, Abel KJ, *et al.*, Complement factor H polymorphism and age-related macular degeneration. *Science*, 2005; 308, 421–4.

Eeles RA, Kote-Jarai Z, Giles GG, *et al.*, Multiple newly identified loci associated with prostate cancer susceptibility. *Nature Genetics*, 2008; 40, 3, 316–21.

Engel LS, Taioli E, Pfeiffer R, *et al.*, Pooled analysis and meta-analysis of glutathione S-transferase M1 and bladder cancer: a HuGE review. *American Journal of Epidemiology*, 2002; 156, 95–109.

Epstein MP, Satten GA, Inference on haplotype effects in case-control studies using unphased genotype data. *American Journal of Human Genetics*, 2003; 73, 1316–29.

Ewen KR, Bahlo M, Treloar SA, *et al.*, Identification and analysis of error types in high-throughput genotyping. *American Journal of Human Genetics*, 2000; 67, 727–36.

Excoffier L, Slatkin M, Maximum-likelihood estimation of molecular haplotype frequencies in a diploid population. *Molecular Biology and Evolution*, 1995; 12, 921–7.

Fan JB, Chee MS, Gunderson KL, Highly parallel genomic assays. *Nature Reviews Genetics*, 2006; 7, 632–44.

Fingerlin TE, Boehnke M, Abecasis GR, Increasing the power and efficiency of disease-marker case-control association studies through use of allele-sharing information. *American Journal of Human Genetics*, 2004; 74, 432–43.

Frayling TM, Timpson NJ, Weedon MN, *et al.*, A common variant in the FTO gene is associated with body mass index and predisposes to childhood and adult obesity. *Science*, 2007; 316, 5826, 889–94.

Frayling TM, Wiltshire S, Hitman GA, *et al.*, Young-onset type 2 diabetes families are the major contributors to genetic loci in the Diabetes UK Warren 2 genome scan and identify putative novel loci on chromosomes 8q21, 21q22, and 22q11. *Diabetes*, 2003; 52, 1857-1863.

Gabriel SB, Schaffner SF, Nguyen H, *et al.*, The structure of haplotype blocks in the human genome. *Science*, 2002; 296, 2225-9.

Gloyn AL, Weedon MN, Owen KR, *et al.*, Large-scale association studies of variants in genes encoding the pancreatic beta-cell KATP channel subunits Kir6.2 (KCNJ11) and SUR1 (ABCC8) confirm that the KCNJ11 E23K variant is associated with type 2 diabetes. *Diabetes*, 2003; 52, 568-72.

Gordon D, Finch SJ, Nothnagel M, *et al.*, Power and sample size calculations for case-control genetic association tests when errors are present: application to single nucleotide polymorphisms. *Human Heredity*, 2002; 54, 22-33.

Goris A, Williams-Gray CH, Foltynie T, *et al.*, No evidence for association with Parkinson disease for 13 single-nucleotide polymorphisms identified by whole-genome association screening. *American Journal of Human Genetics*, 2006; 78, 1088-90

Grant SF, Thorleifsson G, Reynisdottir I, *et al.* Variant of transcription factor 7-like 2 (TCF7L2) gene confers risk of type 2 diabetes. *Nature Genetics*, 2006; 38, 320-32

Groves CJ, Zeggini E, Minton J, *et al.*, Association analysis of 6,736 U.K. subjects provides replication and confirms TCF7L2 as a type 2 diabetes susceptibility gene with a substantial effect on individual risk. *Diabetes*, 2006; 55, 2640-4.

Hageman GS, Anderson DH, Johnson LV, *et al.*, A common haplotype in the complement regulatory gene factor H (HF1/CFH) predisposes individuals to age-related macular degeneration. *Proceedings of the National Academy of Sciences USA*, 2005; 102, 7227-32

Haines JL, Hauser MA, Schmidt S, *et al.*, Complement factor H variant increases the risk of age-related macular degeneration. *Science*, 2005; 308, 409-421

Hirschhorn JN, Lohmueller K, Byrne E, *et al.*, A comprehensive review of genetic association studies. *Genetics in Medicine*, 2002; 4, 45-61.

Hoggart CJ, Clark TG, De Iorio M, *et al.*, Genome-wide significance for dense SNP and resequencing data. *Genetic Epidemiology*, 2008; 32, 2, 179-85.

Hudson TJ, Wanted: regulatory SNPs. *Nature Genetics*, 2003; 33, 439-40.

Hugot JP, Chamaillard M, Zouali H, *et al.*, Association of NOD2 leucine-rich repeat variants with susceptibility to Crohn's disease. *Nature*, 2001; 411, 599-603.

Ioannidis JP, Effect of the statistical significance of results on the time to completion and publication of randomized efficacy trials. *JAMA*, 1998; 279, 281-6.

Ioannidis JP, Gwinn M, Little J, *et al.*, A road map for efficient and reliable human genome epidemiology. *Nature Genetics*, 2006; 38, 1, 3-5.

Ioannidis JP, Ntzani EE, Trikalinos TA, *et al.*, Replication validity of genetic association studies. *Nature Genetics*, 2001; 29, 306-9.

Ioannidis JP, Trikalinos TA, Ntzani EE, *et al.*, Genetic associations in large versus small studies: An empirical assessment. *Lancet*, 2003; 361, 567-71.

Johnson GC, Esposito L, Barratt BJ, *et al.*, Haplotype tagging for the identification of common disease genes. *Nature Genetics*, 2001; 29, 233-7.

Kang SJ, Gordon D, Finch SJ, What SNP genotyping errors are most costly for genetic association studies? *Genetic Epidemiology*, 2004; 26, 132-41.

Keavney B, McKenzie C, Parish S, *et al.*, Large-scale test of hypothesised associations between the angiotensin-converting-enzyme insertion/deletion polymorphism and myocardial infarction in about 5000 cases and 6000 controls. International Studies of Infarct Survival (ISIS) Collaborators. *Lancet*, 2000; 355, 434-42.

Khoury MJ, Little J, Gwinn M, *et al.*, On the synthesis and interpretation of consistent but weak gene-disease associations in the era of genome-wide association studies. *International Journal of Epidemiology*, 2007; 36, 2, 439-45.

Kirk KM, Cardon LR, The impact of genotyping error on haplotype reconstruction and frequency estimation. *European Journal of Human Genetics*, 2002; 10, 616-22.

Klein RJ, Zeiss C, Chew EY, *et al.*, Complement factor H polymorphism in age-related macular degeneration. *Science*, 2005; 308, 385-389

Knapp M, Becker T, Impact of genotyping errors on type 1 error rate of the Haplotype-Sharing Transmission/Disequilibrium Test (HS-TDT). *American Journal of Human Genetics*, 2004; 74, 589-91.

Knight JC, Keating BJ, Rockett KA, *et al.*, In vivo characterization of regulatory polymorphisms by allele-specific quantification of RNA polymerase loading. *Nature Genetics*, 2003; 33, 469-75.

Kraft P, Multiple comparisons in studies of gene x gene and gene x environment interaction. *American Journal of Human Genetics*, 2004; 74, 582-4.

Lander E, Kruglyak L, Genetic dissection of complex traits: guide-lines for interpreting and reporting linkage results. *Nature Genetics*, 1995; 11, 241-247.

Little J, Bradley L, Bray MS, *et al.*, Reporting, appraising, and integrating data on genotype prevalence and gene-disease associations. *American Journal of Epidemiology*, 2002; 156, 300-10.

Lo HS, Wang Z, Hu Y, *et al.*, Allelic variation in gene expression is common in the human genome. *Genome Research*, 2003; 13, 1855-62.

Lohmueller KE, Pearce CL, Pike M, *et al.*, Meta-analysis of genetic association studies supports a contribution of common variants to susceptibility to common disease. *Nature Genetics*, 2003; 33, 177-82.

Loots GG, Ovcharenko I, Pachter L, *et al.*, rVista for comparative sequence-based discovery of functional transcription factor binding sites. *Genome Research*, 2002; 12, 832-9.

Love-Gregory L, Wasson J, Ma J, *et al.*, A common polymorphism in the upstream promoter region of the Hepatocyte Nuclear Factor-4 Gene on Chromosome 20q is associated with Type 2 Diabetes and appears to contribute to the evidence for Linkage in an Ashkenazi Jewish population. *Diabetes*, 2004; 53, 1134-1140

Lykken DT, Statistical significance in psychological research. *Psychological Bulletin*, 1968; 70, 151-9.

Mann V, Hobson EE, Li B, *et al.*, A COL1A1 Sp1 binding site polymorphism predisposes to osteoporotic fracture by affecting bone density and quality. *Journal of Clinical Investigation*, 2001; 107, 899-907.

Mann V, Ralston SH, Meta-analysis of COL1A1 Sp1 polymorphism in relation to bone mineral density and osteoporotic fracture. *Bone*, 2003; 32, 711-7.

Maraganore DM, de Andrade M, Lesnick TG, *et al.*, High-resolution whole-genome association study of Parkinson disease. *American Journal of Human Genetics*, 2005; 77, 5, 685-93.

Marchini J, Cardon LR, Phillips MS, *et al.*, The effects of human population structure on large genetic association studies. *Nature Genetics*, 2004; 36, 512-517

Marron MP, Raffel LJ, Garchon HJ, *et al.*, Insulin-dependent diabetes mellitus (IDDM) is associated with CTLA4 polymorphisms in multiple ethnic groups. *Human Molecular Genetics*, 1997; 6, 1275-82.

McCarthy MI, Progress in defining the molecular basis of type 2 diabetes mellitus through susceptibility-gene identification. *Human Molecular Genetics*, 2004; 13, Suppl 1, R33-41.

McCarthy MI, Smedley D, Hide W, New methods for finding disease-susceptibility genes: impact and potential. *Genome Biology*, 2003; 4, 119.

Mein CA, Barratt BJ, Dunn MG, *et al.*, Evaluation of single nucleotide polymorphism typing with invader on PCR amplicons and its automation. *Genome Research*, 2000; 10, 330-43.

Mitchell AA, Cutler DJ, Chakravarti A, Undetected genotyping errors cause apparent overtransmission of common alleles in the transmission/disequilibrium test. *American Journal of Human Genetics*, 2003; 72, 598-610.

Monsuur AJ, de Bakker PI, Alizadeh BZ, *et al.*, Myosin IXB variant increases the risk of celiac disease and points toward a primary intestinal barrier defect. *Nature Genetics*, 2005; 37, 1341-1344

Niu T, Qin ZS, Xu X, *et al.*, Bayesian haplotype inference for multiple linked single-nucleotide polymorphisms. *American Journal of Human Genetics*, 2002; 70, 157-69.

Nyholt DR, A simple correction for multiple testing for single-nucleotide polymorphisms in linkage disequilibrium with each other. *American Journal of Human Genetics*, 2004; 74, 765-9.

Page GP, George V, Go RC, *et al.*, "Are we there yet?": Deciding when one has demonstrated specific genetic causation in complex diseases and quantitative traits. *American Journal of Human Genetics*, 2003; 73, 711-9.

Palmer LJ, Cardon LR, Shaking the tree: mapping complex disease genes with linkage disequilibrium. *Lancet*, 2005; 366, 9492, 1223-34.

Pe'er I, de Bakker PI, Maller J, *et al.*, Evaluating and improving power in whole-genome association studies using fixed marker sets. *Nature Genetics*, 2006; 38, 663-7.

Pennacchio LA, Olivier M, Hubacek JA, *et al.*, An apolipoprotein influencing triglycerides in humans and mice revealed by comparative sequencing. *Science*, 2001; 294, 169-73.

Power C, Elliott J, Cohort profile: 1958 British birth cohort (National Child Development Study). *International Journal of Epidemiology*, 2006; 35, 1, 34–41.

Redden DT, Allison DB, Nonreplication in genetic association studies of obesity and diabetes research. *Journal of Nutrition*, 2003; 133, 3323–6.

Reich DE, Lander ES, On the allelic spectrum of human disease. *Trends in Genetics*, 2001; 17, 502–10.

Rice TK, Schork NJ, Rao DC, Methods for handling multiple testing. *Advances in Genetics*, 2008; 60, 293–308.

Risch N, Merikangas K, The future of genetic studies of complex human diseases. *Science*, 1996; 273, 1516–1517.

Rubinsztein DC, Easton DF, Apolipoprotein E genetic variation and Alzheimer's disease. a meta-analysis. *Dementia and Geriatric Cognitive Disorders*, 1999; 10, 199–209.

Samani N, Genomewide association analysis of coronary artery disease. *New England Journal of Medicine*, 2007; 357:doi10.1056/nejm0a72366.

Schaid DJ, General score tests for associations of genetic markers with disease using cases and their parents. *Genetic Epidemiology*, 1996; 13, 423–49.

Schaid DJ, McDonnell SK, Wang L, *et al.*, Caution on pedigree haplotype inference with software that assumes linkage equilibrium. *American Journal of Human Genetics*, 2002; 71, 992–5.

Silander K, Mohlke K, Scott L, *et al.*, Genetic variation near the Hepatocyte Nuclear Factor-4 gene predicts susceptibility to Type 2 Diabetes. *Diabetes*, 2004; 53, 1141–1149.

Smyth D, Cooper JD, Collins JE, *et al.*, Replication of an association between the lymphoid tyrosine phosphatase locus(LYP/PTPN22) with type 1 diabetes, and evidence for its role as a general autoimmunity locus. *Diabetes*, 2004; 53, 3020–3033.

Stephens M, Donnelly P, A comparison of bayesian methods for haplotype reconstruction from population genotype data. *American Journal of Human Genetics*, 2003; 73, 1162–9.

Stephens M, Smith NJ, Donnelly P, A new statistical method for haplotype reconstruction from population data. *American Journal of Human Genetics*, 2001; 68, 978–89.

Storey JD, Tibshirani R, Statistical significance for genomewide studies. *Proceedings of the National Academy of Sciences USA*, 2003; 100, 9440–5.

Stram DO, Tag SNP selection for association studies. *Genetic Epidemiology*, 2004; 27, 365–74.

Tabor HK, Risch NJ, Myers RM, Opinion: Candidate-gene approaches for studying complex genetic traits: practical considerations. *Nature Reviews Genetics*, 2002; 3, 391–7.

Teng J, Risch N, The relative power of family-based and case-control designs for linkage disequilibrium studies of complex human diseases. II. Individual genotyping. *Genome Research*, 1999; 9, 234–41.

Thomas H, Jaschkowitz K, Bulman M, *et al.*, A distant upstream promoter of the HNF-4alpha gene connects the transcription factors involved in maturity-onset diabetes of the young. *Human Molecular Genetics*, 2001; 10, 2089-97.

Ueda H, Howson JM, Esposito L, *et al.*, Association of the T-cell regulatory gene CTLA4 with susceptibility to autoimmune disease. *Nature*, 2003; 423, 506-11.

Wacholder S, Chanock S, Garcia-Closas M, *et al.*, Assessing the probability that a positive report is false: an approach for molecular epidemiology studies. *Journal of the National Cancer Institute*, 2004; 96, 434-442

Weedon MN, Schwarz PE, Horikawa Y, *et al.*, Meta-analysis and a large association study confirm a role for calpain-10 variation in type 2 diabetes susceptibility. *American Journal of Human Genetics*, 2003; 73, 1208-12.

Weinberg CR, Methods for Detection of Parent-of-Origin Effects in Genetic Studies of Case-Parents Triads. *American Journal of Human Genetics*, 1999; 65, 229-235.

Weiss KM, Clark AG, Linkage disequilibrium and the mapping of complex human traits. *Trends in Genetics*, 2002; 18, 19-24.

Wellcome Trust Case Control Consortium, Genome-wide association study of 14,000 cases of seven common diseases and 3,000 shared controls. *Nature*, 2007; 447, 7145, 661-78.

Wright AF, Hastie ND, Complex genetic diseases: controversy over the Croesus code. *Genome Biology*, 2001; 2, comment 2007.1-2007.8.

Zareparsi S, Branham KE, Li M, *et al.*, Strong association of the Y402H variant in complement factor H at 1q32 with susceptibility to age-related macular degeneration. *American Journal of Human Genetics*, 2005, 88, 149-53

Zeggini E, Rayner W, Morris AP *et al.* An evaluation of HapMap sample size and tagging SNP performance in large-scale empirical and simulated data sets. *Nature Genetics*, 2005; 37, 1320-2

Ziegler A, Konig IR, Thompson JR, Biostatistical aspects of genome-wide association studies. *Biom J*, 2008; 50, 1, 8-28.

Zondervan KT, Cardon LR, The complex interplay among factors that influence allelic association. *Nature Reviews Genetics*, 2004; 5, 89-100.

Zondervan KT, Cardon LR, Designing candidate gene and genome-wide case-control association studies. *Nature Protocols*, 2007; 2, 10, 2492-501.

SIX

Biobanks and biobank harmonisation

Paul R. Burton, Isabel Fortier, Mylene Deschênes, Anna Hansell, Lyle J. Palmer

Summary

Over the past decade and a half, genetic epidemiology has experienced an important shift from family-based studies of genetic linkage to individual-based studies of genetic association (Chapters One-Four). In part, this follows the recognition that if the 'common disease, common variant hypothesis'[1-5] is true for at least a proportion of important genetic determinants of complex disease, these determinants – which will predominantly exhibit weak aetiological effects[6] – will be identified more easily using association studies of population-based samples[7]. The shift to using association studies has been accompanied by an increasing methodological focus on optimal approaches to the design, analysis, meta-analysis and reporting of genetic association studies[8-15; 65-67] (www.cdc.gov/genomics/hugenet/strega.htm). This chapter describes these changes, and the growing international focus on biobanks with which they are associated.

Introduction

Although some association studies are undertaken using family-based designs[16; 17], the majority of contemporary association studies involve the recruitment of unrelated individuals into either case-control or cohort studies[6; 17; 18] (see also Chapters Three and Five). If the aim is to study a single disease and to explore associations between that disease and one or more genetic variants, a case-control study is generally more cost effective[19; 20]. Most simple disease-gene association studies are therefore based on case-control studies[6; 15; 17; 18]. However, cohort studies also offer a number of distinct advantages[21-24]. Their principal benefit is that cohort studies – and *only* cohort studies – enable a full range of exposure and outcome information to be collected *prospectively*. If assessment is undertaken retrospectively, both systematic and random errors are more likely to distort the measurement of pre-morbid lifestyle and environment and their observed relationships with disease. Retrospective designs are more susceptible not only to various forms of information bias and selection bias, but also to bio-clinically mediated reverse causality. This latter arises when a disease state influences a supposed 'exposure' – for example, when the early symptoms of coronary artery disease persuade a sufferer to stop smoking and to change their diet. Prospective cohort studies are not entirely immune from these same errors and biases, but they are generally less susceptible than are case–control studies[21-23].

Until recently (Manolio *et al.* 2008; Hindorff *et al.* 2009), and regardless of the epidemiological design that was adopted, genetic association studies exhibited a persistent and serious lack of consistency[10; 12; 18; 25-29]. The repeated failure to replicate positive results was ascribed[10; 13-15; 25; 28; 30] to a wide variety of different problems including: insufficient sample size; inadequately rigorous tests of statistical significance; extreme biological and phenotypic complexity; measurement error; sub-structure in population ancestry; and effect–size bias. It was also recognised that such problems were compounded by between–investigator and between–study heterogeneity in: study design; analytic methods; phenotype definition; genetic structure; linkage disequilibrium; the choice of genetic markers that were genotyped and environmental exposures that were measured.

In responding to these issues, it was recognised that nothing could be done about the intrinsic 'complexity' of the 'complex' diseases and that the only reasonable line of attack was therefore to modify those characteristics of study design and analysis that could be controlled. As also discussed in Chapter 3, the principal avenues of attack were seen as being: to use rigorous p-values to strictly limit the type 1 error; to greatly increase the 'actual' sample size by designing larger studies; to augment the 'effective' sample size by enhancing the quality of design and analysis of individual studies (including an emphasis on obtaining objective biological measures, rather than relying solely on potentially subjective questionnaire responses, and on reducing measurement error and other forms of misassessment); and to focus on the robust replication of positive findings using a variety of high quality studies with different designs[9; 11; 17; 18; 27; 28; 31-34; 65].

In the event, two major strategies were adopted widely. These have greatly enhanced our ability to detect and replicate phenotype-genotype associations. The first involved the development and widespread use of genotyping chips to support genome wide association studies (GWAS) characterising hundreds of thousands of SNPs. There is no doubt that a series of major studies using these chips has accounted for the striking recent progress that has been made in detecting genetic associations with complex diseases (Manolio *et al.* 2008; Burton *et al.* 2009): "in the past three years genome–wide association studies (GWAS) .... have reproducibly identified hundreds of associations of common genetic variants with over 80 diseases and traits (www.genome.gov/gwastudies)" (Hindorff *et al.* 2009). But, it is also important to recognise that although the use of GWAS chips with increasing coverage has undoubtedly increased statistical power: "marked differences in genome coverage may not translate into appreciable differences in power and that, when taking budgetary considerations into account, the most powerful design may not always correspond to the chip with the highest coverage" (Spencer *et al.* 2009). In fact, it can reasonably be argued that it is the marked increase in sample size and the enhancement of study design (e.g. improved quality of measurement) which has accompanied the introduction of GWAS chips that has been primarily responsible for a marked increase in statistical power and that it is this that has led to our improved recent success. This is the second major strategy that has been adopted, and across the world, it is this that has been responsible for the investment of substantial resources in the design and implementation of large-scale biobanks[22]. These are the focus of Chapter 6.

Biobanks are so called because they involve the systematic storage of biological material (such as blood or extracted DNA) and information from a large number of participants. Biobanks may be disease-specific, exposure-oriented or population-based[35]. Many are being set up de novo as large genomic studies including the UK Biobank[69] (www.ukbiobank.ac.uk), the Joondalup Family Health Study (www.jfhs.org.au) and LifeGene (www.thepersonalgenome.com/2005/02/swedish_lifegen.html). Others, such as the 1958 Birth Cohort[36] and the Million Women Study[37] were originally conceived as conventional epidemiology studies and were later transformed to enable genomic analysis by collecting DNA samples and obtaining appropriate consents from the study participants. A comprehensive list of biobanks with at least 10,000 subjects is maintained by the Public Population Program in Genomics (P[3]G; www.p3gobservatory.org); as of August 2009 there were 136 independent studies in the catalogue.

Disease-specific biobanks

Disease-specific biobanks collect material and information from subjects that have already developed a particular disease. Tumour banks provide a good example in the oncology field[35]. Such biobanks represent resources both for research and to guide the clinical management of individual patients. The 'case' members of a large case–control study incorporating the collection of biological samples might also be considered to form a disease-specific biobank[38], as may an extensive set of affected relatives from a genetic linkage study[39]. Finally, some therapeutic clinical trials involve the systematic collection and storage of information and biological material on substantial numbers of patients with a particular disease. Such a trial can also be viewed as generating a disease-specific biobank[40].

Exposure-oriented biobanks

Exposure-orientated biobanks recruit subjects sharing a common exposure. These include occupational biobanks (for example, www.ymed.lu.se/eng/research.html) and the biobanks that are sometimes initiated after potentially dangerous environmental exposures[41] (http://rarediseases.info.nih.gov/html/reports/fy2004/niehs.html).

Population-based biobanks

A population-based biobank is an epidemiological study that collects and stores biological material and information from generally healthy participants recruited from a demographically or geographically defined population. Most commonly, such biobanks are cross-sectional or cohort studies that recruit unrelated individuals (P[3]G Observatory), although some are based on the recruitment of families[42] or twins[43]. The controls in a population-based case-control study can also form the basis of a population-based biobank (www.wtccc.org.uk/), as can the recruits in a preventative clinical trial carried out in healthy participants[44].

There is therefore nothing particularly new about the modern concept of biobanks. The only departure from long-standing epidemiological tradition is the sheer size of the largest initiatives now being proposed and the strong emphasis that is placed on obtaining biological material and a broad range of phenotypic information (P[3]G Observatory). That said, although the fundamental epidemiological changes are relatively minor, there has been a substantial change in the national and international context in which such studies are now being developed. In consequence, the addition of genomic data to large-scale epidemiological studies now presents a number of major scientific, logistic, ethical and political challenges (www.p3g.org). This has important implications for the design, conduct and exploitation of biobanks.

Population-based cohort biobanks

Population-based cohort biobanks can conveniently be divided into two main categories. Those in the first category set out to study the aetiological architecture of dichotomous disease-related traits (such as diabetes [yes/no] or lung cancer [yes/no]). These biobanks must be very large in order to provide adequate statistical power (for example, UK Biobank and LifeGene)[22-24; 45]. Biobanks in the second category focus on deep phenotyping. That is, they aim to undertake an intensive and high-quality assessment of relevant exposures and outcomes (for example, the Avon Longitudinal Study of Parents and Children[46]). The emphasis of deep phenotyping is often placed on quantitative measures. Such a measure may either represent an endpoint in its own right (such as a behavioural score) or an intermediate (endophenotype) on a biological pathway that potentially links determinants with disease (for example insulin resistance in a study of diabetes[46]). The statistical power associated with the analysis of quantitative traits is generally higher than that associated with dichotomous traits. Therefore the required sample size for biobanks in the second category can then be markedly smaller than that required for those in the first category[33; 47].

Population-based cohort biobanks can fulfil several important scientific roles: studies of the joint effects of genes and environment; exposure-based studies; and studies of the aetiological determinants of disease progression.

Studies of the joint effects of genes and environment

Nested case-control studies, based on cohorts, that focus on dichotomous disease end-points provide an ideal platform for the comprehensive study of the *joint* effects of genes and environment or lifestyle. Similarly, in a deeply phenotyped cohort, the joint relationship can be explored between a quantitative disease-related trait, genetic determinants and lifestyle or environmental factors. In either setting, a cohort design is essential if scientific interest focuses on lifestyle/ environment determinants that cannot reliably be assessed retrospectively[22; 23]. When the prospective assessment of environment/lifestyle is not mandatory, an association analysis based on a cohort study can make use of the prevalent cases of a disease that are present at recruitment, as well as the incident cases that arise later. In UK Biobank, for example, it is estimated[45] that among the 500,000 participants aged between 40 and 69 at recruitment, more than 10,000 will have diabetes, more than 7,000 will have ischaemic heart disease and more than 1,500 will have Parkinson's disease.

Exposure-based studies

In a nested case-control study, subgroups of a cohort are sampled on their disease status, and diseased cases and healthy controls are then compared on the basis of their exposure to genetic and/or environmental determinants. In contrast, an exposure-based study involves sampling a cohort on the basis of exposure status and then comparing disease-related traits between the subgroups defined by the differential exposure. As the potentially expensive assessment of the disease related traits is restricted solely to those relatively few participants that have been sampled into the exposure-defined subgroups, this type of study provides a highly cost effective way to undertake intensive investigation of aetiological determinants and causal pathways in a cohort study. In a very large population-based cohort, even rare exposures will usually be present in sufficient numbers to allow a powerful analysis. The exposure of interest will often be a genotype or a haplotype, and such studies may then be called genotype-based studies. The extent to which these will ultimately become a central feature of the research to be undertaken on population-based biobanks will be determined by the cost of genotyping. If the cost falls to such an extent that comprehensive genotyping of a whole cohort becomes a practical and affordable reality, genotype-based studies are set to become as important as nested case-control studies. Given dramatic reductions in the cost of genotyping[18], this may well occur.

The aetiological determinants of disease progression

Because cohort studies allow the ongoing and repeated assessment of key phenotypes and exposures, they provide an ideal platform for studies of the genetic and environment or lifestyle determinants of disease progression.

As a vehicle for research involving the aetiological determinants of a complex disease, a population-based cohort offers additional advantages too. Firstly, provided the required disease outcomes are carefully assessed, a single cohort can support the study of many different diseases[23]. In consequence, a single well designed cohort study might actually be more cost effective than a series of disease-specific case-control studies. Secondly, a population-based cohort study enables replication and validation studies of putative disease-determinant associations to be undertaken in a population that can be mapped demographically onto the general population. This can be crucial when it is important to know whether a putative disease-determinant association has important implications for the broader public health[34]. Thirdly, because the cost is likely to be prohibitive, a cohort study would not usually be adopted as the design of choice for investigating the simple association between a disease and a genetic variant. However, once a large cohort has been set up for one or more of the reasons considered above, the marginal cost associated with also using it to provide a platform to support the investigation of such associations might be very low. Fourthly, a large population-based cohort study can provide an ideal sampling frame from which to recruit a set of 'common controls' that may be used as the comparison group – for genetic case-control analyses – for a set of cases generated by any disease arising in that same population base.

How large is large?

Given the emphasis that is increasingly being placed on adequate sample size[22; 23; 24; 33; 45; 47], how large do population-based biobanks really need to be? For a cohort biobank focusing on dichotomous disease traits, sample size is usually determined by the statistical power requirements of the nested case-control studies that will be based on it. In other words, statistical power is not fixed by the size of the cohort as a whole, but by the number of cases of the disease of interest that will arise in that cohort[22; 45]. Power calculations undertaken for UK Biobank indicate that, even under ideal circumstances, if 80% power is required to detect small direct effects, such as an odds ratio in the range 1.20-1.30 associated with a binary exposure (genetic or environmental) that has a population prevalence between 10% and 25%, at least 5,000 cases of the disease of interest are needed[45]. Here, ideal circumstances include the requirements that there is no misclassification error, that the scientific focus is on evaluating the association between a complex disease and one or more candidate genes, and that the statistical significance defined can be $p < 0.0001$. An absolute minimum of 5,000 cases is also required to provide 80% power to detect an interaction effect of moderate size (for example an interaction odds ratio in the range 1.5 to 2.0 between two binary exposures, each with a population prevalence between 10% and 25%). Other commentators have also recommended that there should be an attempt to accrue at least 5,000 cases of a disease of interest[24]. However, if appropriate account is also taken of the misclassification of exposures and outcomes as well as the impact of unmeasured aetiological determinants, formal simulation-based power calculations indicate that the desirable sample size rises to at least 10,000 to 20,000 disease cases[45], or sometimes even more[68].

The statistical power considerations described in the preceding paragraph are as pertinent to a conventional case-control study as to a nested case-control analysis based on a cohort study. There are several ways to accrue such a large number of cases. (i) A co-ordinated infrastructure to support large case-control studies could be constructed. (ii) A large prospective cohort study could be set up, and the required number of incident cases could be recruited. (iii) Research groups around the world might work together to harmonise biobanks (both pre-existing and planned) to allow the pooling of information between them (P[3]G Observatory)[14; 15]. In keeping with a rational strategy to maintain the flexibility of the scientific infrastructure to optimally support biomedical research, all three approaches are being developed simultaneously.

Large case-control initiatives

In the UK, the MRC DNA Network (www.dnabank.mrc.ac.uk/) included 13 extensive series of cases of a variety of important complex diseases. Following on from this, the Wellcome Trust Case Control Consortium took 2,000 cases from each of eight complex diseases (some from the MRC network) and compared them with 3,000 common controls generated by combining a set of 1,500 geographically representative controls sampled from the 1958 Birth Cohort and an equivalent number from a national sample of blood transfusion donors (WTCCC)[70; 71]. In the United States the Genetic Association Information Network (GAIN) initiative is setting up a network of large case-control studies involving 1,000 to 3,000 cases of each disease (www.genome.gov/17516722)[72]. Commercial biotechnology companies are also active in this area. For example, in order to provide an infrastructural resource to support case-control studies, Affymetrix set up a web-based pool of common controls all genotyped using the Affymetrix 500K chip (www.affymetrix.com/products/arrays/specific/genome_wide/control_cohort.affx).

Large population-based cohort biobanks

Table 6.1 presents examples of the largest population-based biobanks that are already in existence or are in the later phases of planning (P[3]G Observatory).

The two criteria for inclusion in the table are that the designated project has enrolled, or intends to enrol, a minimum of 100,000 (generally) healthy participants and that there is an intention to collect both conventional epidemiological information and biological material, the latter in a form that permits the extraction of DNA and will therefore support genetic/genomic analysis. Among the biobanks listed, five have recruited, or intend to recruit, at least 500,000 participants (Table 6.1).

In order to demonstrate some of the typical features of a large cohort-based biobank, UK Biobank can be used as a convenient illustrative example. It is to be a multipurpose research platform that will recruit 500,000 middle-aged volunteers (40-69 years) of both sexes from across Great Britain, recruitment to the main study commenced in May 2007[69; 73], and, as of July 2009, 340,000 participants have

Table 6.1: Large population-based research biobanks (planned and current)

Name	Design	Sample size	Country	Age at recruitment (years)		Current status	URL
				Min	Max		
European Prospective Investigation into Cancer and Nutrition (EPIC)	Cohort	520,000	Denmark, France, Greece, Germany, Italy, Netherlands, Norway, Spain, Sweden and United Kingdom	30	70	Follow-up	www.iarc.fr/epic
UK Biobank	Cohort	500,000	United Kingdom	40	69	Pilot	www.ukbiobank.ac.uk
Kadoorie Study of Chronic Disease in China (KSCDC)	Cohort	500,000	China	35	74	Recruitment; follow-up	www.ctsu.ox.ac.uk/~kadoorie/public
LifeGene	Cohort	500,000	Sweden	-	55	Preparation	
Cancer Prevention Study 3 (CPS-3)	Cohort	500,000	United States	30	65	Pilot	www.cancer.org/docroot/RES/RES_6_6.asp
Cancer Prevention Study II Nutrition Cohort (CPS)	Cohort	184,200	United States	50	74	Follow-up	www.cancer.org/docroot/RES/content/RES_6_2_Study_Overviews.asp?
LifeLines	Cohort	165,000	Netherlands	Various		Preparation	www.umcg.nl/azg/nl/english/nieuws/83575
NUgene	Cohort	100,000	United States	18	-	Preparation	www.nugene.org/
ProtecT Study	Cohort	120,000	United Kingdom	50	69	Recruitment; follow-up	www.epi.bris.ac.uk/protect/index.htm
Singapore Consortium of Cohort Studies	Cohort	250,000	Singapore	21	65	Pilot	

Table 6.1: continued

Name	Design	Sample size	Country	Age at recruitment (years) Min	Max	Current status	URL
Danish National Birth Cohort	Birth cohort	100,000	Denmark	At birth		Follow-up	www.serum.dk/sw9314.asp
National Children's Study	Birth cohort	100,000	United States	At birth		Pilot	www.nationalchildrensstudy.gov
Norwegian Mother and Child Cohort Study	Birth cohort	100,000	Norway	At birth		Recruitment; follow-up	www.fhi.no/artikler/?id = 51488
Estonian Genome Project	Cohort	100,000	Estonia	18	-	Pilot	www.geenivaramu.ee
JANUS Project	Cohort	600,000	Norway	20	-	Follow-up	www.medisin.ntnu.no/ism/nofe/norepid/ne_2006_1/2006(1)%2011-Gislefoss.pdf
GenomEUtwin	Twin cohorts	>600,000	Finland, Sweden, Norway, Denmark, the Netherlands and Italy, United Kingdom and Australia	Various		Follow-up	www.genomeutwin.org
Prostate, Lung, Colorectal and Ovarian Cancer Screening Trial (PLCO)	Clinical trial	154,938	United States	55	74	Follow-up	www.cancer.gov/prevention/plco/index.html
The Environmental Determinants of Diabetes in the Young (TEDDY) Study	Child cohort	220,800	United States, Germany, Sweden and Finland	At birth		Recruitment; follow-up	http://teddy.epi.usf.edu/TEDDY/index.htm
Joondalup Family Health Study	Cohort	80,000	Australia	Various		Pilot	www.jfhs.org.au

been enrolled (www.ukbiobank.ac.uk/about/backing/celeb.php). Recruitment is population-based rather than disease- or exposure-based, and the aim is to recruit participants from across the full breadth of British society. However, it is not intended that the UK Biobank will be demographically representative – in a rigorous epidemiological sense – of the general population of Great Britain. Social, demographic, exposure and health data will be collected via questionnaire and from a physical examination. Blood will be taken and stored as a source of DNA and for the purposes of biomarker-based exposure and phenotype assessment. Once recruited, the state of health of individual participants will be monitored via the health care information systems and, in particular, new cases of significant complex disease will be identified. A substantial component (though not all) of the important research involving UK Biobank will be based on nested case-control studies. An important implication is that because incident cases of disease will be identified from the routine information systems that necessarily hold restricted details and are subject to non-negligible misclassification error, appropriate investment will have to be made in validating and classifying the cases that are to be used in the nested studies.

Harmonising biobanks

The need, or not, for biobank harmonisation will be determined principally by the extent to which individual (stand-alone) biobanks can answer the important scientific questions that need to be addressed over the next few decades. It was earlier argued that if scientific interest focuses on the aetiological architecture of a dichotomous complex disease state, at least 10,000-20,000 cases of that disease are required in order to provide adequate statistical power to detect realistic relative risks[45;] Can any individual biobank – either disease-based or population-based – be large enough to provide a research infrastructure of this nature?

It is true that a small number of case-control studies (such as in the ISIS study of myocardial infarction[38]) do contain this number of cases, but the great majority do not. Even national case-control initiatives such as the Wellcome Trust Case-Control Consortium and GAIN that are widely perceived as being 'very large' include markedly fewer than 10,000 cases. It would therefore appear that, unless case-control studies are going to become much larger in the future, harmonisation and pooling of such studies is ultimately going to be essential[14; 15].

Consider the alternative option: how large does a cohort biobank need to be in order to generate 10,000 to 20,000 cases of a disease of scientific interest? The response to this question depends on many things[22; 23; 45]. These include the particular disease that is of scientific interest; the age at recruitment of the cohort; the particular population being recruited and its underlying rates of disease; the effectiveness of the longitudinal tracking that will identify the incident cases of disease; and many others. However, even before considering these factors, it is important to note that the original question is inadequately specified. The number of cases is a function not only of the size of the cohort, but also of the length of follow-up. It is true that the size of a cohort places a finite upper bound on the number of cases that can potentially be generated (if everybody in the cohort is followed-up until their death). If the required number of cases falls below that bound, then the question becomes 'How long is it reasonable to wait?'

Table 6.2 provides indicative answers to these questions, based on the expected rate of generation of incident cases of a number of key complex diseases in UK Biobank[22; 45]. The expected times to each threshold for each specific disease are based on computer-generated simulations of the longitudinal evolution of UK Biobank that take appropriate account of the age range at recruitment and the likely duration of the recruitment phase of the study. They are based on published age- and sex-specific incidence and death rates in the UK[45]. A simulated participant is considered to be no longer at risk of becoming an incident case of a particular disease once he/she has died, or if he/she has already developed that disease. Appropriate account is taken of the fact that participants in cohort studies tend to be unusually healthy. For the specific purposes of the analyses underlying the construction of Table 6.2, it is also assumed that the proportion of participants that are prepared to remain in active contact with UK Biobank over time will be similar to the profile of ongoing retention of follow-up in the 1958 Birth Cohort Study (www.cls.ioe.ac.uk/studies.asp?section = 000100020003) and the Whitehall Study[48].

Manolio has published corresponding, and generally very consistent, estimates based on data from the United States[23]. Consequently, although Table 6.2 and the text refer to the expected generation of incident cases in one particular biobank,

Table 6.2: The expected rate of accrual of incident cases of selected complex diseases

	Time (years) to achieve:				
	1,000 cases	2,500 cases	**5,000 cases**	10,000 cases	20,000 cases
Non-cancers:					
MI and coronary death	2	4	5	8	14
Diabetes mellitus	2	3	5	7	11
Chronic obstructive pulmonary disease (COPD)	4	6	9	14	27
Rheumatoid arthritis	7	15	36	-	-
Cancers:					
Breast cancer (F)	4	7	11	19	-
Colorectal cancer	6	10	15	25	-
Lung cancer	7	13	22	-	-
Stomach cancer	17	36	-	-	-

The expected time in years after the commencement of recruitment by which UK Biobank (500,000 recruits aged 40-69 years) will have generated the specified number of cases of selected complex diseases[22; 45]. The expected times take appropriate account of the fact that participants in cohort studies tend to be healthier than the general population. They also assume that the proportion of participants that are prepared to remain in active contact with the study over time will be similar to the profile of ongoing retention of follow-up in the 1958 Birth Cohort Study (www.cls.ioe.ac.uk/studies.asp?section=000100020003) and the Whitehall Study[48].

it seems entirely reasonable to claim that two robust conclusions may be drawn and might reasonably be considered to apply to any cohort biobank:

- It is only the commonest of complex diseases that will ever generate 10,000–20,000 cases, even in a very large cohort biobank that recruits as many as 500,000 participants. For example, even though lung cancer is far from being a rare condition, UK Biobank will never generate as many as 10,000 cases, even if all participants are followed throughout their remaining life.
- Even for those conditions that are common enough to generate as many as 10,000–20,000 cases in a cohort of size 500,000, the wait will generally be measured in decades. For example, it will take 27 years to generate 20,000 cases of chronic obstructive pulmonary disease.
- In addition, it can realistically be argued that it is beyond the capacity of most national funding bodies to properly finance a cohort that is much larger than 500,000 participants.

International harmonisation of biobanks

In light of the discussion in the previous section, it seems not unreasonable to conclude that the only way to amass a large enough number of cases of many of the important complex diseases – inside a reasonable time frame and at an affordable cost – is to supplement the setting up of large case–control and cohort biobanks with a concerted international effort to promote harmonisation and data integration between biobanks. Indeed, it can be argued that this is both scientifically and politically essential if governments, funding agencies and the general public are to be reassured that the huge international investment that is currently being made in population-based biobanking is being wisely directed.

With minor modification, biobank harmonisation has been defined (Alastair Kent, personal communication) as: 'A set of procedures that promote, both now and in the future, the effective interchange of *valid* information and samples between a number of studies or biobanks, accepting that there may be important differences between those studies'. In other words, it encompasses any activity that helps to ensure that study design, scientific methods, research tools and systems for the acquisition, storage and transmission of data, samples and phenotypes are not only fit for their original purpose, but also enhance the interchange of information, samples and other related information between studies – within the ethical, legal and technical constraints that necessarily apply.

The major collaborative enterprise implied by a strategy to actively promote biobank harmonisation, and thereby to facilitate data integration, offers a number of clear scientific benefits. Firstly, it will allow the investigation of diseases, such as stomach cancer (Table 6.2) and ovarian cancer[45], that are certainly not viewed as rare, but are not common enough to ever generate as many as 5,000 cases in a cohort study including 500,000 participants. Secondly, it will enable critical analyses to be undertaken earlier. Thirdly, data pooling will support the study of weaker associations between aetiological determinants and common diseases. Fourthly, it will enable powerful analyses based on subgroups defined, for example, by age, sex or ethnicity or by subtypes of the disease of interest (such as thrombotic stroke). Lastly, the synthesis of information from cohort studies from around the world allows at least the potential to investigate the impact of a much broader range of lifestyles, thereby increasing the power to detect joint effects of genes and environment.

It is possible to distinguish between two approaches to harmonisation. These may be designated 'prospective harmonisation' and 'retrospective harmonisation'. Prospective harmonisation is aimed at modifying study design and conduct, ahead of time, in order to render the subsequent data and sample pooling more efficient and more straightforward. Retrospective harmonisation is aimed at pooling data, samples and phenotypes that have already been collected, in studies with unavoidably heterogeneous designs. In an ideal world, all biobanks would be optimally designed from the perspective of prospective harmonisation. In other words, their design and proposed conduct would take appropriate account of the need to collect and store data and samples in a way that enhanced the prospects of future data sharing both generically (for example, the development and use of a common core set of questionnaire variables that are shared by most or many biobanks) and specifically (for example, the use of a more extensive set of common questionnaire variables and measurements to be collected by a small group of biobanks that deliberately set out to be mutually harmonised).

Optimisation of the design, conduct, analysis and exploitation of individual biobanks involves a complex interplay between bioscience, social science, ethics, law and politics. It is not therefore surprising that there are a series of essential conditions that must be met before it is possible to even contemplate integration of data between biobanks. These conditions include a requirement that: each individual biobank is of a high enough scientific quality; study designs and data item definitions are compatible, or can be rendered compatible; an appropriate ethical and legal framework ·is in place; there is an agreed oversight process that enables access to the required data and samples; the concept of harmonisation and integration is supported by *all* relevant stake-holders; and collaboration between researchers is real and meaningful.

Many biobanks collect sensitive information and monitor health and exposure status over a very long period of time. Furthermore, most of the research questions that will ultimately be addressed cannot possibly be specified when participants are initially recruited into a biobank and their consent is formally obtained. The sensitivity of the information collected, combined with uncertainty about its potential use, creates a major challenge to traditional models of consent and demands a redefinition of the ethical and legal frameworks currently in use.

The normative landscape is also a challenge. There has been a burgeoning of laws, ethical guidelines and rules governing population genomics, especially with respect to the protection of privacy. Moreover, the lack of a common taxonomy has created confusion, especially in an international context. Making sense of this normative complexity is a major challenge for collaborative projects[49]. In this context, one might be tempted to hope for a 'one size fits all' framework to simplify the process of international collaboration. But agreement on a common normative framework can be built only on proper respect for cultural differences and values. The creation of a common international approach to ethical standards can be undertaken only when local values and legal specificities are taken into appropriate account.

At present, there is a worldwide move to facilitate access to raw data in a manner that preserves appropriate protections for participants and researchers. Many leading international organisations have underscored the importance of sharing, in a pre-competitive manner. For example, one such organisation has said 'Open access to publicly funded data provides greater returns from the public investment in research, generates wealth through downstream commercialisation of outputs and provides decision makers with facts needed to address complex often transnational problems'[50].

The underlying culture of competition in science undoubtedly stimulates research, but it also causes some resistance to full collaboration. If such collaboration is to be successful, researchers must be given the flexibility to develop their own research interests and must be reassured that their intellectual property will be protected. Yet international success stories of collaboration, such as the Human Genome Project[51], the International HapMap Project[52] and the Wellcome Trust Case Control Consortium [5,6] have clearly demonstrated the feasibility of these major international projects and the tremendous scientific impact that they can have.

There are several groups around the world that are already advancing harmonisation programs for population-based research biobanks. These include the EPIC study (Table 6.1) that was designed from the outset as a harmonised group of cohort studies running in ten separate European countries[53], and GenomEUtwin[54] (www.genomeutwin.org/). At a higher integrative level, at least two international groups have been focusing specifically on the harmonisation of population-based biobanks across the world. These include the P^3G^{34} (P^3G) and PHOEBE (Promoting Harmonisation of Epidemiological Biobanks in Europe). Furthermore, the Human Genome Epidemiology Network (HuGENet) provides an internationally accessible forum that represents 'a collaboration of individuals and organisations committed to the assessment of the impact of human genome variation on population health and how genetic information can be used to improve health and prevent disease'[15] (www.cdc.gov/genomics/hugenet/default. htm)[74-76].

Conclusions

Genetic knowledge will be useful in the clinical arena only if it can be placed in an appropriate epidemiological and medical/public health context[55-59]. The principal purpose of the science to be underpinned by biobanks is to extend our knowledge of the causal mechanisms linking aetiological determinants to disease and disease progression[22]. It is knowledge of these mechanisms that will ultimately lead to new diagnostic, preventative and therapeutic interventions that will have an important impact on clinical medicine and on the health of the public. An important implication of this philosophy is that, as in Mendelian randomisation[22; 77], associations with genetic determinants that have a small population-attributable risk or a small relative risk can nevertheless provide important information about causal pathways that may lead to the development of interventions that have a major impact on the public health.

The major payoffs from individual biobanks based on a prospective cohort design are unlikely to occur before the second or third decades after recruitment [22; 23; 45]. That said, there might be some quick wins. For example, cross-sectional analyses based on common binary or quantitative phenotypes at recruitment (for example, type 2 diabetes or spirometry-based measures of lung function) will allow powerful population-based replication, or non-replication, of genetic associations previously identified in non-representative subpopulations. Similar opportunities will exist for certain questions in pharmacogenetics[60; 61]. But the implementation of research findings in clinical practice is slow and can take a decade or more[62]. It is important that biomedical and public health scientists avoid overstating the pace at which returns can realistically be expected.

The rate of progress on all fronts will be greatly accelerated by active initiatives aimed at harmonising biobanks. There has been substantial recent investment in international biobank harmonisation under initiatives including the P³G funded by Genome Canada and Genome Quebec and PHOEBE, funded by the European Union under Framework 6. P³G is an international umbrella organisation for population-based biobanks. Its aims are: to foster collaboration between biobanks; to optimise the design, set-up and research activity of population-based biobanks; to promote harmonisation; to facilitate transfer of knowledge to advance public health; and to provide training. PHOEBE works in close collaboration with P³G but has a focused remit to explore, describe and push forward opportunities for biobanks and biobank harmonisation across Europe. This investment provides good grounds for optimism that the science of biobanking is set to move forward rapidly. It may be anticipated that there will be an ever-increasing quality of individual biobanks and a rapidly expanding capacity for harmonisation and data pooling.

Although they are not without controversy[63; 64], it is now widely accepted[22-24; 34; 45] that large genetic cohort studies have an important role to play in furthering our understanding of complex human disease. In the face of significant uncertainty about how best to proceed with the discovery of genes for complex human disease and how best to make use of the discoveries that are made, it is important to emphasise that *everything* in human genetics is context-specific. There is no one study design or analytic approach that will be optimal in all circumstances. It is clear that a flexible, multi-faceted approach is desirable. If scientific progress is to be optimised, genetic cohort studies, case-control studies and family studies will all be needed. Each individual design has its own scientific niche – the optimal design is always specific to the particular scientific question being asked. That said, it is becoming increasingly obvious that, with very few exceptions, *any* study designed to investigate the aetiology of a complex disease will necessarily be very large and it is equally clear that we must take all opportunities to harmonise and integrate data between biobanks.

Acknowledgements

The international biobank harmonisation program of P^{3}G is funded by Genome Canada and Genome Quebec. The methodological research and educational program in genomic epidemiology at the University of Leicester is also supported by the programs of: PHOEBE (Promoting Harmonization of Epidemiological Biobanks in Europe) funded by the European Union under the Framework 6 program; MRC Cooperative Grant G9806740, Program Grant 00\3209 from the National Health and Medical Research Council (NHMRC) of Australia, and by Leverhulme Research Interchange Grant F/07134/K. A. Hansell is a Research Fellow funded by the Wellcome Trust. This work was supported in part by the Wind-over-Water Foundation (to L.J. Palmer).

References

1. Lander ES, The new genomics: Global views of biology, *Science*, 1996; 274, 5287, 536-9.
2. Reich DE, Lander ES, On the allelic spectrum of human disease. *Trends in Genetics*, 2001; 17, 9, 502-10.
3. Pritchard JK, Cox NJ, The allelic architecture of human disease genes: common disease-common variant...or not? *Human Molecular Genetics*, 2002; 11, 20, 2417-23.
4. Hirschhorn JN, Lohmueller K, Byrne E, *et al.*, A comprehensive review of genetic association studies. *Genetics in Medicine*, 2002; 4, 2, 45-61.
5. Lohmueller KE, Pearce CL, Pike M, *et al.*, Meta-analysis of genetic association studies supports a contribution of common variants to susceptibility to common disease. *Nature Genetics*, 2003; 33, 2, 177-82.
6. Hattersley AT, McCarthy MI, What makes a good genetic association study? *Lancet*, 2005; 366, 9493, 1315-23.
7. Risch N, Merikangas K, The future of genetic studies of complex human diseases. *Science*, 1996; 273, 1516-1517.
8. Silverman EK, Palmer LJ, Case-Control Association Studies for the Genetics of Complex Respiratory Diseases. *American Journal of Respiratory Cell and Molecular Biology*, 2000; 22, 6, 645-648.
9. Dahlman I, Eaves IA, Kosoy R, *et al.*, Parameters for reliable results in genetic association studies in common disease. *Nature Genetics*, 2002; 30, 2, 149-50.
10. Cardon LR, Bell JI, Association study designs for complex diseases. *Nature Reviews Genetics*, 2001; 2, 2, 91-9.

11. Zondervan KT, Cardon LR, The complex interplay among factors that influence allelic association. *Nature Reviews Genetics*, 2004; 5, 2, 89-100.

12. Goldstein DB, Ahmadi KR, Weale ME, *et al.*, Genome scans and candidate gene approaches in the study of common diseases and variable drug responses. *Trends in Genetics*, 2003; 19, 11, 615-22.

13. Little J, Khoury MJ, Bradley L, *et al.*, The human genome project is complete. How do we develop a handle for the pump? *American Journal of Epidemiology*, 2003; 157, 8, 667-73.

14. Ioannidis JP, Gwinn M, Little J, *et al.*, A road map for efficient and reliable human genome epidemiology. *Nature Genetics*, 2006; 38, 1, 3-5.

15. Little J, Higgins JPT, *The HuGENet™ HuGE Review Handbook, version 1.0*: www.hugenet.ca. 2006.

16. Hopper JL, Bishop DT, Easton DF, Population-based family studies in genetic epidemiology. *Lancet*, 2005; 366, 9494, 1397-406.

17. Cordell HJ, Clayton DG, Genetic association studies. *Lancet*, 2005; 366, 9491, 1121-31.

18. Palmer LJ, Cardon LR, Shaking the tree: mapping complex disease genes with linkage disequilibrium. *Lancet*, 2005; 366, 9492, 1223-34.

19. Breslow NE, Day NE, *Statistical Methods in Cancer Research. Volume 1 - The analysis of case-control studies*. Lyon: International Agency for research on Cancer, 1980.

20. Rothman K, Greenland S, *Case-control studies*. Philadelphia: Lippincott-Raven, 1998:93-114.

21. Breslow NE, Day NE, *Statistical Methods in Cancer Research. Volume 2 - The design and analysis of cohort studies*. Lyon: International Agency for Research on Cancer, 1987.

22. Davey Smith G, Ebrahim S, Lewis S, *et al.*, Genetic epidemiology and public health: hope, hype, and future prospects. *Lancet*, 2005; 366, 9495, 1484-98.

23. Manolio TA, Bailey-Wilson JE, Collins FS, Genes, environment and the value of prospective cohort studies. *Nature Reviews Genetics*, 2006; 7, 10, 812-20.

24. Collins FS, The case for a US prospective cohort study of genes and environment. *Nature*, 2004; 429, 6990, 475-7.

25. Ioannidis JP, Ntzani EE, Trikalinos TA, *et al.*, Replication validity of genetic association studies. *Nature Genetics*, 2001; 29, 3, 306-9.

26. Lohmueller KE, Pearce CL, Pike M, *et al.*, Meta-analysis of genetic association studies supports a contribution of common variants to susceptibility to common disease. *Nature Genetics*, 2003; 33, 2, 177-82.

27. Tabor HK, Risch NJ, Myers RM, Opinion: Candidate-gene approaches for studying complex genetic traits: practical considerations. *Nature Reviews Genetics*, 2002; 3, 5, 391-7.

28. Weiss KM, Terwilliger JD, How many diseases does it take to map a gene with SNPs? *Nature Genetics*, 2000; 26, 2, 151-7.

29. Terwilliger JD, Goring HH, Gene mapping in the 20th and 21st centuries: statistical methods, data analysis, and experimental design. *Human Biology,* 2000; 72, 1, 63-132.

30. Risch NJ, Searching for genetic determinants in the new millennium. *Nature,* 2000; 405, 6788, 847-56.

31. Goldstein DB, Tate SK, Sisodiya SM, Pharmacogenetics goes genomic. *Nature Reviews Genetics,* 2003; 4, 12, 937-47.

32. Thomas DC, Clayton DG, Betting odds and genetic associations. *Journal of National Cancer Institute,* 2004; 96, 6, 421-3.

33. Wong MY, Day NE, Luan JA, *et al.,* The detection of gene-environment interaction for continuous traits: should we deal with measurement error by bigger studies or better measurement? *International Journal of Epidemiology,* 2003; 32, 51-57.

34. Khoury MJ, Millikan R, Little J, *et al.,* The emergence of epidemiology in the genomics age. *International Journal of Epidemiology,* 2004; 33, 936-944.

35. Husebekk A, Iversen O-J, Langmark F, *et al., Biobanks for Health - Report and Recommendations from an EU workshop.* Oslo: Technical report to EU Commission, 2003.

36. Power C, Elliott J, Cohort profile: 1958 British birth cohort (National Child Development Study). *International Journal of Epidemiology,* 2006; 35, 1, 34-41.

37. Beral V, Bull D, Reeves G, Endometrial cancer and hormone-replacement therapy in the Million Women Study. *Lancet,* 2005; 365, 9470, 1543-51.

38. Clarke R, Xu P, Bennett D, *et al.,* Lymphotoxin-alpha gene and risk of myocardial infarction in 6,928 cases and 2,712 controls in the ISIS case-control study. *PLoS Genetics,* 2006; 2, 7, e107.

39. Samani NJ, Burton P, Mangino M, *et al.,* A genomewide linkage study of 1,933 families affected by premature coronary artery disease: The British Heart Foundation (BHF) Family Heart Study. *American Journal of Human Genetics,* 2005; 77, 6, 1011-20.

40. The ATBC Cancer Prevention Study Group, The alpha-tocopherol, beta-carotene lung cancer prevention study: design, methods, participant characteristics, and compliance. *Annals of epidemiology,* 1994; 4, 1-10.

41. Dubrova YE, Bersimbaev RI, Djansugurova LB, *et al.,* Nuclear weapons tests and human germline mutation rate. *Science,* 2002; 295, 5557, 1037.

42. Palmer LJ, Knuiman MW, Divitini ML, *et al.,* Familial aggregation and heritability of adult lung function: results from the Busselton Health Study. *European Respiratory Journal,* 2001; 17, 4, 696-702.

43. Ferreira MA, O'Gorman L, Le Souef P, *et al.,* Variance components analyses of multiple asthma traits in a large sample of Australian families ascertained through a twin proband. *Allergy,* 2006; 61, 2, 245-53.

44. Oddy WH, Holt PG, Sly PD, *et al.,* Association between breast feeding and asthma in 6 year old children: findings of a prospective birth cohort study. *British Medical Journal,* 1999; 319, 7213, 815-9.

45. Burton PR, Hansell A, *UK Biobank: the expected distribution of incident and prevalent cases of chronic disease and the statistical power of nested casecontrol studies*. Manchester, UK: UK Biobank Technical Reports, 2005.

46. Shultis WA, Leary SD, Ness AR, *et al.*, Haemoglobin A(1c) is not a surrogate for glucose and insulin measures for investigating the early life and childhood determinants of insulin resistance and Type 2 diabetes in healthy children. An analysis from the Avon Longitudinal Study of Parents and Children (ALSPAC). *Diabetic Medicine,* 2006; 23, 12, 1357-63.

47. Luan JA, Wong MY, Day NE, *et al.*, Sample size determination for studies of gene-environment interaction. *International Journal of Epidemiology,* 2001; 30, 5, 1035-40.

48. Clarke R, Breeze E, Sherliker P, *et al.*, Design, objectives, and lessons from a pilot 25 year follow up re-survey of survivors in the Whitehall study of London Civil Servants. *Journal of Epidemiology and Community Health,* 1998; 52, 6, 364-9.

49. Knoppers BM, Saginur M, The Babel of genetic data terminology. *Nature Biotechnology,* 2005; 23, 8, 925-7.

50. Working group for OECD, International framework to promote access to data. Adopted by OECD: Declaration on access to research data from public funding, Jan 30th, 2004 (item 8): OECD, 2003.

51. International Human Genome Sequencing Consortium. Finishing the euchromatic sequence of the human genome. *Nature,* 2005; 431, 931-45.

52. The International HapMap Project. The International HapMap Project. *Nature,* 2003; 426, 6968, 789-96.

53. Gormally E, Hainaut P, Caboux E, *et al.*, Amount of DNA in plasma and cancer risk: A prospective study. *International Journal of Cancer,* 2004; 111, 5, 746-749.

54. Harris JR, Willemsen G, Aitlahti T, *et al.*, Ethical issues and GenomEUtwin. *Twin Research,* 2003; 6, 5, 455-63.

55. Khoury MJ, McCabe LL, McCabe ER, Population screening in the age of genomic medicine. *New England Journal of Medicine,* 2003; 348, 1, 50-8.

56. Burke W, Genomics as a probe for disease biology. *New England Journal of Medicine,* 2003; 349, 10, 969-74.

57. Merikangas KR, Risch N, Genomic priorities and public health. *Science,* 2003; 302, 5645, 599-601.

58. Kelada SN, Eaton DL, Wang SS, *et al.*, The role of genetic polymorphisms in environmental health. *Environmental Health Perspective,* 2003; 111, 8, 1055-64.

59. Shostak S, Locating gene-environment interaction: at the intersections of genetics and public health. *Social Science and Medicine,* 2003; 56, 11, 2327-42.

60. Israel E, Chinchilli VM, Ford JG, *et al.*, Use of regularly scheduled albuterol treatment in asthma: genotype-stratified, randomised, placebo-controlled cross-over trial. *Lancet,* 2004; 364, 9444, 1505-12.

61. Roses AD, Pharmacogenetics. *Human Molecular Genetics,* 2001; 10, 20, 2261-7.

62. Rosenberg RN, Translating biomedical research to the bedside: a national crisis and a call to action. *JAMA,* 2003; 289, 10, 1305-6.

63. Clayton D, McKeigue PM, Epidemiological methods for studying genes and environmental factors in complex diseases. *Lancet,* 2001; 358, 9290, 1356-60.

64. Highfield R, £62m Biobank may not be worth it, says Professor. *Daily Telegraph,* 2004; 8.

65. Chanock SJ, Manolio T, Boehnke M, *et al.* Replicating genotype-phenotype associations. *Nature* 2007; 447 (7145): 655-60.

66 Trikalinos TA, Salanti G, Zintzaras E, Ioannidis JP. Meta-analysis methods. *Adv Genet* 2008; 60: 311-34.

67. Ziegler A, Konig IR, Thompson JR. Biostatistical aspects of genome-wide association studies. *Biom J* 2008; 50 (1): 8-28.

68 Burton PR, Hansell AL, Fortier I, *et al.* Size matters: just how big is BIG?: Quantifying realistic sample size requirements for human genome epidemiology. *Int J Epidemiol* 2008.

69. Palmer LJ. UK Biobank: bank on it. *Lancet* 2007; 369 (9578): 1980-2.

70. Wellcome Trust Case Control Consortium, Genome-wide association study of 14,000 cases of seven common diseases and 3,000 shared controls. *Nature* 2007; 447 (7145): 661-78.

71. Burton PR, Clayton DG, Cardon LR, *et al.* Association scan of 14,500 nonsynonymous SNPs in four diseases identifies autoimmunity variants. *Nat Genet* 2007; 39 (11): 1329-37.

72. Manolio TA, Rodriguez LL, Brooks L, *et al.* New models of collaboration in genome-wide association studies: the Genetic Association Information Network. *Nat Genet* 2007; 39 (9): 1045-51.

73. Jackson C, Best N, Elliott P, UK Biobank Pilot Study: stability of haematological and clinical chemistry analytes. *Int J Epidemiol* 2008; 37 Suppl 1: i16-22.

74. Smith GD, Gwinn M, Ebrahim S, Palmer LJ, Khoury MJ. Make it HuGE: human genome epidemiology reviews, population health, and the IJE. *Int J Epidemiol* 2006; 35 (3): 507-10.

75. Khoury MJ, Little J, Gwinn M, Ioannidis JP. On the synthesis and interpretation of consistent but weak gene-disease associations in the era of genome-wide association studies. *Int J Epidemiol* 2007; 36 (2): 439-45.

76. Zintzaras E, Lau J. Trends in meta-analysis of genetic association studies. *J Hum Genet* 2008; 53 (1): 1-9.

77. Ebrahim S, Davey Smith G, Mendelian randomization: can genetic epidemiology help redress the failures of observational epidemiology? *Hum Genet* 2008; 123 (1): 15-33.

SEVEN

Population health aspects of genetic epidemiology: genomic profiling, personalised medicine and Mendelian randomisation

George Davey Smith, Shah Ebrahim, Sarah Lewis, Lyle J. Palmer

Summary

The recent advances covered in this book have equipped genetic epidemiologists with powerful tools for studying the genetic architecture of complex diseases and have resulted in a cornucopia of new genetic discoveries. However, the direct contribution to public health of new genomic knowledge is difficult to discern. The major focus has been on attempts to use known genetic variants to identify individuals at high risk of disease, coupled with appropriate management to reduce their risk[1]. The potential of pharmacogenomic studies to contribute to personalised medicine has also been widely heralded[2-4; 163; 164]. In this chapter we briefly review these approaches and conclude that major contributions to either health care or public health have yet to be made. More encouraging are findings from association studies of well-characterised genetic variants that are being used to strengthen causal inferences about modifiable environmental exposures – sometimes referred to as 'Mendelian randomisation'[5-14]. These are offering powerful new methods for observational epidemiology to study modifiable environmental exposures.

Genomic profiling in the prevention and treatment of common diseases

Since the launch of the human genome project the potential of using genetic knowledge to contribute to improving human health has been widely championed[15-17; 163; 164]. In a striking image from his 1999 Shattuck lecture, Francis Collins described a hypothetical consultation in 2010 with John, a 23-year-old man. This patient has a high cholesterol level following screening and undergoes extensive genetic testing[18]. Table 7.1 shows the hypothetical genotypes found and his relative risks of the relevant diseases, which are impressively worrying. These indicate 2.5- and 6-fold increased risks of coronary heart disease and lung cancer, respectively.

Table 7.1a: Results of genetic testing in a hypothetical patient in 2010

Condition	Genes involved *	Relative risk (current estimate)	Lifetime risk (%)
Reduced risk			
Prostate Cancer	HPC1, HPC2, HPC3	0.4	7
Alzheimer's disease	APOE, FAD3, XAD	0.3	10
Elevated risk			
Coronary heart disease	APOB, CETP	2.5	70
Colon cancer	FCC4, APC	4.0	23
Lung cancer	NAT2	6.0	40

* *HPC1, HPC2*, and *HPC3* are the three genes for hereditary prostate cancer; *APOE* is the gene for apolipoprotein E; *FAD3* and *XAD* are hypothetical genes for familial Alzheimer;s dementia; *APOB* is the gene for apolipoprotein B; *CETP* is the gene for cholesteryl ester transfer protein; *FCC4* is the hypothetical gene for familial colon cancer; *APC* is the gene for adenomatous polyposis coli; and *NAT2* is the gene for N-acetyltransferase 2.

Source: Collins, 1999[18]

Table 7.1b: Results of genetic testing in a hypothetical patient in 2010 (from Collins, 1999) and updated estimates of relative risks associated with common variants in these genes in brackets (see Box 1)

Condition	Genes involved*	Relative risk (current estimate)	Lifetime risk (%)
Reduced risk			
Prostate Cancer	HPC1, HPC2, HPC3	0.4 **(1)**	7
Alzheimer's disease	APOE	0.3 **(0.3)**	10
Elevated risk			
Coronary heart disease	APOB, CETP	2.5 **(1)**	70
Colon cancer	APC	4.0 **(1)**	23
Lung cancer	NAT2	6.0 **(1)**	40

* HPC1, HPC2, and HPC3 are the three genes for hereditary prostate cancer; APOE is the gene for apolipoprotein E; FAD3 and XAD are hypothetical genes for familial Alzheimer;s dementia; APOB is the gene for apolipoprotein B; CETP is the gene for cholesteryl ester transfer protein; FCC4 is the hypothetical gene for familial colon cancer; APC is the gene for adenomatous polyposis coli; and NAT2 is the gene for N-acetyltransferase 2.

Source: Adapted from Collins, 1999

Box 7.1: Fate of genetic variants advocated for screening in 2010

It is instructive to consider how evidence regarding the genetic variants advocated for screening in Francis Collins' Shattuck lecture (Table 7.1) have fared over the past 10 years.

The patient, John, was said to be at elevated risk of coronary artery disease because of variants in his cholesterol ester transfer protein (*CETB*) and apolipoprotein B (*APOB*) genes). Variants in the *CETP* and *APOB* were said to identify a relative risk of coronary heart disease of 2.5, based on small studies up to that date. The CETP Taq1b variant has been extensively investigated, and a recent meta-analysis suggests a per-allele odds ratio for coronary heart disease of 1.05 (95% CI 1.01 to 1.09)[149]. For common variation in APOB the best current estimate is a per-allele effect of 1.10 (95% CI 1.03 to 1.18)[150].

A striking relative risk of 6.0 was given in Collins' table for lung cancer risk among smokers for variants in the *NAT2* gene, again based on small studies. A case-control study of 2,500 participants reported an equivalent odds ratio of 0.96 (95% CI: 0.79 to 1.16), a null effect that has subsequently been seen in other studies[151; 152]. The phenomenon whereby small genetic association studies show large effect sizes that are not replicated in larger studies is well recognised[126; 127]; similarly, the association between a genetic polymorphism and disease has been shown to be stronger in the first study than in subsequent research[127].

One gene for which a sizeable complex disease risk does appear to be realised is the association of the *APOE* gene with Alzheimer's disease, although a recent cohort study of individuals found that the *APOE* ε4 allele acts as a risk factor for Alzheimer's disease by accelerating onset, but has a more modest effect on lifetime susceptibility[128]. In a further recent study the relative risk of Alzheimer's disease among individuals heterozygous for ε4 was 1.4 (95% CI: 1.0 to 2.0) and among ε4 homozygotes was 3.1 (95% CI: 1.6 to 5.9)[129]. The importance of APOE variation in Alzheimer's disease has been recently reiterated in a genome-wide association study[153]. As for the other genes listed in Collins' table, rare mutations in these genes have been shown to confer very high risk among a small number of families, but little or no increased risk in the general population. For example, the *ELAC* gene, which lies in the *HPC2* region, was identified as being linked to prostate cancer in family studies. A recent meta-analysis of two common polymorphisms in the *ELAC* gene[130] reported ORs of 1.04 (95% CI: 0.50 to 1.09) for Leu217 homozygotes and 1.18 (95% CI: 0.98 to 1.42) for Thr541 homozygotes and heterozygotes combined. The meta-analysis also showed that the largest and most recent study showed no effect associated with either polymorphism.

Rare mutations in *APC* are related to colon cancer risk, but at the time of Collins' Shattuck lecture a report of a large risk associated with a common variant, E1317Q, had recently appeared[131]. However, a subsequent case-control study of colorectal cancers demonstrated no association between this variant in an analysis comparing cases with spouse controls (OR 0.83, 95% CI: 0.31 to 2.26). The investigators concluded that E1317Q '…does not appear to confer an increased risk for colorectal neoplasia in the general population. Genetic screening for E1317Q is not indicated'[132].

Despite the fact that one of the few genes for which a sizeable complex disease risk does appear to be realised is the *APOE* gene, in 1995 the American College of Medical Genetics and American Society of Human Genetics stated that it did not recommend that the *APOE* gene be used for routine diagnosis or predictive testing for Alzheimer's disease, because this genotype did not provide sufficient sensitivity and specificity to allow it to be used as a test [133].

Unsurprisingly in this future scenario, three of the 11 variants were fictional names for unknown variants of a type that Collins predicted would be identified by 2010. So what was the impact of the eight variants that were already known in 1999? Box 7.1 summarises the post-1999 fate of the predictive power of these variants, and demonstrates that, with few exceptions, later evidence suggests that they are related to much smaller – if any – increased risks of disease, and would not be of value within a routine battery of genetic tests applied during medical consultations.

Although Box 7.1 makes it clear that the story with respect to Collins' variants looks rather negative and, in general, genetic epidemiology has yet to fulfil its promise in this respect, there are a few success stories. A meta-analysis of the association between the complement factor H Y402H polymorphism and age-related macular degeneration found a robust association, with an approximately sixfold increase in risk among CC homozygotes at the appropriate codon in the gene versus TT homozygotes[19]. This particular variant is thought to have a population-attributable risk of around 40%. Finding 'an elephant in the ballroom' – an increase in risk of such magnitude – is rare, and it is now widely acknowledged that in most cases we can expect to see more modest increases (relative risks of around 1.1 to 1.5) in risk associated with any particular common variant, with correspondingly low population-attributable risks. However, as knowledge in this area is growing fast, it may become increasingly possible to categorise individuals according to the number of 'at risk' alleles they have for several genetic variants, which alone are associated with relative risks in the 1.1 to 1.3 range, identifying groups with a more substantially increased risk of disease. There are now robustly replicated associations between common variants in 11 genes and type 2 diabetes risk – however, these variants explain less than 10% of the overall risk of disease, even when combined[165]. Furthermore, once it is possible to identify high-risk individuals, the question then becomes 'what does one do with this information?' Thus, although recent discoveries have advanced our understanding of population-level susceptibility to diseases such as type 2 diabetes, the proportion of risk explained at present is generally too small for effective clinical translation in terms of screening or individualised prevention. Adding the common variants associated with type 2 diabetes into predicted algorithms makes very little, if any, contribution to prediction above that provided by conventional clinical measures[154; 155].

The genetic variants themselves do not point to any particular forms of preventive treatment and could serve only as levers to increase the motivation for lifestyle changes that would also have benefits (albeit less in absolute terms) for those carrying low-risk genotypes. Thus, in the case of a genetic variants and lung cancer risk discussed by Collins, even if a variant was identified that was associated with a considerably larger risk of lung cancer among smokers, it could have adverse consequences if identifying such genetic risk led others to believe that they could smoke with impunity, which would not be the case. Identification of susceptibility in the population could have negative consequences for the uptake of health promotion advice that is beneficial for all, irrespective of genotype, and paradoxically could lead to increased risk in the population.

Do we simply have to wait a bit longer to achieve Collins' vision of 'genetically based, individualised preventive medicine'? In a recent editorial Collins and colleagues have reiterated their belief in personalised genomic medicine, and

Box 7.2: Criteria for appraising the viability, effectiveness and appropriateness of a screening programme, adapted for genetic screening tests, from UK National Screening Committee guidelines [134]

The disorder
- The disorder should be an important health problem.
- The epidemiology and natural history of the disorder should be adequately understood and there should be detectable genetic risk factors.
- A limited number of mutations in the responsible gene(s) within the target population should be responsible for a high proportion of the genetic risk.
- The detectable genetic mutations or polymorphisms should have high penetrance.
- All the cost-effective primary prevention interventions should have been implemented as far as practicable.

The test
- There should be a simple, safe, precise and validated genetic screening test.
- The test should be acceptable to the population.
- There should be an agreed policy on the further diagnostic investigation of individuals with a positive test result and on the choices available to those individuals.

The treatment
- There should be an effective treatment or intervention for patients identified as being at risk through genetic testing, with evidence of early treatment consequent on the results of genetic testing leading to better outcomes than late treatment initiated after risk becomes evident for other reasons, such as the development of symptoms.
- There should be agreed evidence-based policies covering which individuals should be offered treatment and the appropriate treatment to be offered.
- Clinical management of the condition and patient outcomes should be optimised by all health care providers before participation in a screening programme.

The screening programme
- There must be evidence from high-quality randomised controlled trials that the genetic screening programme is effective in reducing mortality or morbidity.
- There should be evidence that the complete genetic screening programme is clinically, socially and ethically acceptable to health professionals and the public.
- The benefit from the genetic screening programme should outweigh the physical and psychological harm.
- The opportunity cost of the screening programme should be economically balanced in relation to expenditure on medical care as a whole (value for money).
- There should be a plan for managing and monitoring the screening programme and an agreed set of quality assurance standards.

- Adequate staffing and facilities for testing, diagnosis, treatment and programme management should be made available before the commencement of the screening programme.
- All other options for managing the condition should have been considered.
- Evidence-based information, explaining the consequences of testing, investigation and treatment, should be made available to potential participants to assist them in making an informed choice.
- Public pressure for widening the eligibility criteria for the genetic screening test should be anticipated.

updated their scenario (this time with 'Amy' instead of 'John') from 2010 to 2020. They do note that in the recent past such a 'scenario of personalized medicine in routine clinical care would have seemed wildly optimistic'. For genomic profiling to have a role in public health, the technology should be evaluated explicitly using accepted standards of evidence applied to any screening programme (Box 7.2). When judged against these criteria most proposed genetic screening tests would fail, because either the excess risk borne by a carrier of the variant is too low, identification would not point to use of an acceptable treatment, or it would not influence an already supported management strategy.

Genetic screening

Common complex diseases are our focus, as these have the greatest influence on population health, but we will briefly discuss other modalities of molecular genetic screening. Genetic screening can be of several basic types – recessive carrier screening, recessive disease screening, autosomal dominant disease screening, pharmacogenetic risk screening, employment risk screening and complex genetic disease screening (see Table 7.2 for examples)[20].

Table 7.2: Categories of molecular genetic risk screening

Type	Disease, gene or exposure
Recessive carrier screening	Cystic fibrosis, Ashkenazi-Jewish screening panel
Recessive disease screening	Hereditary haemochromatosis
Autosomal dominant disease screening	*BRCA1/BRCA2*
Pharmacogenetic risk screening	Malignant hypothermia
Employment risk screening	N-acetyl transferase and occupational exposure to arylamines
Complex genetic disease screening	Methylane tetrahydrofolate reductase, angiotensin-1-converting enzyme

Source: Adapted from [20]

The aim of population screening for genetic diseases, both recessive and dominant, is to detect individuals at high risk of developing a particular disease for which early detection and or treatment will lead to a better prognosis.

Recessive carrier screening aims to identify couples who are at risk of having children affected by a recessive disease. This intervention therefore facilitates prenatal diagnosis and informed choice regarding abortion. Cystic fibrosis has been a major focus of such screening, particularly since the US National Institutes of Health Consensus Development Conference in 1997 recommended that couples seeking prenatal care should be offered such a service[21]. This recommendation was echoed by the American College of Obstetricians and Gynaecologists and the American College of Medical Genetics in 2001[22; 23]. A panel of mutations that lead to defective cystic fibrosis transmembrane conductance regulator (CFTR) protein are screened for, with the most common of the 1,000 or so identified mutations being included[24]. Such testing is now very widespread in the US[25], but doubts remain about the accuracy and selection of the tests[25; 26], and unexpected complexity in the genotype-phenotype relationships have emerged[27]. There are also concerns regarding the cost-effectiveness of such screening[26] and the potential psychosocial consequences of a widespread counselling and screening service[28-32].

Screening strategies for particular population of origin groups, such as Ashkenazi-Jewish populations[33; 34], with predisposition to rare diseases due to rare recessive variants have been developed. Populations derived from small founder groups, such as the Finnish population[35], are at increased risk of rare hereditary diseases and characterisation of their rare mutations could be used for screening[36].

Recessive disease screening aims at detecting homozygotes or compound heterozygotes at increased but modifiable risk of disease. For example, hereditary haemochromatosis is a common autosomal recessive disorder, present at around one in 300 in European-origin populations[37], in which increased iron absorption results in excessive accumulation[37]. This disease meets many of the guidelines for population screening in that it is primarily caused by a single mutation in the *HFE* gene[38; 39], and around 80% of patients are homozygous for a single mutation, C282Y[38], that can be easily, accurately and inexpensively detected. A second variant, H63D, may increase the risk of haemochromatosis among individuals with a single copy of the C282Y mutation, although the effects of the H63D mutation are less well understood[40]. Symptoms are severe and non-specific, but early diagnosis and treatment improves prognosis[40]. The current clinical approach is to search for haemochromatosis in the presence of clinical disease such as kidney failure, although such patients will already have irreversible complications. The College of American Pathologists have stated that screening is warranted for all people over the age of 20, but recommended phenotypic (iron overload) testing rather than genotypic screening[41], because a negative test for C282Y homozygosity does not rule out disease due to other mutations. There is also growing uncertainty surrounding the penetrance of the common mutation. Thus, even for haemochromatosis – seen as the paradigmatic example of a disease for which genetic screening had major potential[42] – considerable doubts remain. For other widely discussed conditions – for example, risk of venous thromboembolism in relation to factor V Leiden and prothrombin variants – the case for molecular genetic screening is even weaker[43], although a recent large-scale meta-analysis of individual studies has demonstrated strong evidence for their association with cardiovascular diseases[44].

Autosomal dominant disease screening identifies individuals who have inherited one or two copies of a dominant disease allele and are therefore at high risk of developing the disease. Around 5% of women who develop breast cancer have a strong hereditary predisposition to the disease, with multiple family members affected, often at an early age[45]. Mutations in one of two genes, *BRCA1* and *BRCA2*, are responsible for susceptibility in most of these 'breast cancer families', and women with a least one copy of these mutations are also at increased risk for several other cancers, particularly ovarian cancer. *BRCA* gene mutations are highly penetrant, although penetrance appears to be dependent on the strength of family history and is probably a consequence of the severity of the mutation[46]. It is therefore difficult to predict lifetime risk and hence to offer relevant advice. Studies have found that among carriers opting for prophylactic mastectomy, the number of life years gained compared with those who opted for surveillance alone was just 2.9 years among those with a low-penetrance mutation[47]. Population-wide screening using *BRCA1/2* mutations is technically difficult and expensive, given that many of the mutations in *BRCA1* and *BRCA2* are fairly specific. In the UK, many clinical genetics services screen only individuals with a strong family history[48], because as in all autosomal dominant diseases of high penetrance it is highly likely that other family members will be affected. Therefore, screening by family history is likely to be more cost effective than genotyping as an initial step.

Pharmacogenetic risk screening Certain individuals exhibit severe drug reactions as a result of mutations in genes involved in drug metabolism or drug receptors, and identifying individuals with such mutations prior to treatment could avoid adverse effects[1; 2]. For some rare conditions there are developments that could be of benefit; for example, a rare variant in the *TPMT* gene identifies children with acute leukaemia at risk for severe side effects to mercaptopurine[49]. For most more widely used pharmacological agents there is little currently indicated pharmacogenetic screening. Consider malignant hyperthermia, a rare but life-threatening condition occurring as a result of exposure to anaesthetics and depolarising muscle relaxants in genetically susceptible individuals[50]. Although a high proportion of disease cases are autosomal dominant, having a mutation in just one copy of the ryanodine receptor gene[50] many different disease-causing mutations have been identified. This makes screening difficult and expensive at the moment[1; 2]. Nearly all known examples of pharmacogenetic tests relate to adverse reactions to therapy, rather than magnitude of response to therapy. We are, however, beginning to see some excellent examples of well-validated pharmacogenetic genes that predict adverse responses and that have changed (and will continue to change) clinical practice. For instance, hypersensitivity reaction to abacavir (a commonly used anti-retroviral agent in HIV treatment) is strongly associated with the presence of the *HLA-B*5701* allele and was introduced into clinical practice in Western Australia in 2004. A recent double-blind, prospective, randomised study involved 1956 patients from 19 countries definitely established the effectiveness of prospective *HLA-B*5701* screening to prevent the abacavir hypersensitivity reaction, and showed that a pharmacogenetic test can be used to prevent a specific toxic effect of a drug. Similarly, common genetic variation predicting adverse responses to statins[156] and flucloxacillin[157] have recently appeared. Pharmacological agents are in general evolutionarily novel exposures, therefore even marked adverse responses to them will not have been under the influence of selection. Thus they may provide one of the currently rare examples of substantial gene-by-environment interaction.

Employment risk screening aims to detect people who are susceptible to specific workplace exposures, allowing them to avoid exposure and reduce their risk. For example, the enzyme *N*-acetyltransferase is involved in the metabolism of various chemical substances including arylamines, which are used in dry cleaning and other industries. These have been shown to cause cancers, in particular bladder cancer [51]. However, in common with most mutations, the relative risk of cancer is small in genetically susceptible individuals, and all individuals will generally benefit from a reduced exposure to carcinogens. The risk of disease associated with exposure tends to be greater than the risk associated with genotype[51], making primary prevention through limiting exposure the intervention of choice. There are fears that employers might use genetic screening in preference to primary prevention, and such testing could lead to employment discrimination according to genotype, although at present employment risk screening is little used.

Genetic variation and susceptibility to common diseases

The contribution of genetic epidemiology to an evidence base for conventional genetic screening has not yet delivered an appreciable number of implementable targets, as outlined earlier. However, it is often suggested that the greatest potential benefit from genomic profiling would be in improving common disease prevention. Currently, though, there is still a long road ahead from discovery to translation into clinical or public health practice[52]. The main problem is that although we now have a large number of validated variants associated with susceptibility to common diseases, there are very few common genetic variants that are known to *substantially* increase the risk of common diseases (Box 7.1). Where polymorphisms, which increase disease risk, have been identified, interventions are generally framed in terms of advice to reduce exposure to lifestyle factors that are, in any case, the target of interventions. Thus, the hypothetical John, described by Collins, was told that he had six times the risk of lung cancer compared with other smokers, because of his genotype. Although a common variant affecting risk of lung cancer has recently been identified (in the *CHRNA5* gene)[166; 167] the associated relative risk of lung cancer adjusted for tobacco smoking was small.

Furthermore, the variant appears to influence lung cancer risk through influencing the ability to quit smoking[158] and, among smokers, inhalation patterns[159]. Even non-susceptible individuals who smoke are at high preventable risk of lung cancer (and other common diseases), so it would be most effective to apply smoking cessation programs to the whole population. Evidence that genetic test results can motivate behavioural change is currently lacking[52]. Indeed there is the potential problem that people identified as being at lower risk of lung cancer if they continue smoking than are other smokers may be less inclined to quit following such genomic profiling.

New, confirmed associations between genetic variants and increased disease risk may not have an impact on prevention strategies. For example, the *MTHFR* 677TT genotype may increase coronary artery disease risk by around 20% relative to the 677CC genotype[53; 54], and testing for this variant to prevent heart disease risk has been advocated[55]. However, if this genotype does increase coronary artery disease risk, it does so by increasing homocysteine levels, which can be lowered by folate supplementation. Within each genotype group there will be wide variations in homocysteine levels as there are several polymorphisms in other genes, together with environmental factors, that determine blood homocysteine. Less than 2% of the variability in homocysteine is explained by the C667T polymorphism of the *MTHFR* gene[56]. Genotyping only one variant will give a less sensitive prediction of risk than that given by simply measuring homocysteine levels. As Humphries *et al*[43] state, 'for a genetic test to be useful in the management of CVD [cardiovascular disease] it must have predictive powers over and above accepted risk factors that can easily be measured, usually inexpensively and with high reproducibility and replicability.' Folate supplementation has been recommended as a component of the 'polypill' to reduce cardiovascular risk in all individuals over the age of 55, irrespective of genotype. However, more recent evidence has cast doubt on the whole story, with the demonstration that *MTHFR* 677TT genotype coronary artery disease association is null in United States and European studies[57], and the publication of a growing number of negative randomised clinical trials of folate supplementation.

Behavioural and physiological risk factors show considerable clustering, such that people with one adverse factor (such as elevated cholesterol) are more likely to have others (such as obesity, insulin resistance or smoking), generating high risk of disease, and consequently provide useful tools for targeting interventions[58]. This clustering arises because social processes or underlying states such as obesity, by necessity, generate such interrelationships. By contrast, the possession of one risk–increasing genetic variant will generally be independent of others, such that the proportion of the population bearing several variants associated with moderate risk, that together could produce substantial elevated risk, would be very small. This is illustrated by an example from type 2 diabetes – a combination of known risk alleles was associated with a sixfold risk of diabetes, but this combination was present in only 1% of the population. Khoury *et al.*[59] show that overall reduction in disease burden based on population intervention, regardless of genotype, will generally be more substantial than intervention targeted according to genotype.

Currently, asking about family history is probably the best tool we have in terms of 'genetic screening' of the general population, and perhaps we should be concentrating on this, rather than pursuing a shopping list of currently favoured polymorphisms that have modest effects on disease risk[60; 61]. However, this has not stopped an apparently lucrative business of offering genetic profiling for complex disease by many internet–based companies[160].

Personalised medicine: hype or hope?

The use of genetic variants as screening tests overlaps with, but is distinct from, the notion of personalised medicine, in which it is envisaged that precise treatment protocols will depend on genotypic information. Our concern in this chapter is with common germline genetic variants that might influence choice of therapeutic regime for disease prevention or treatment of common disease, rather than the identification of genes expressed in rare diseases that aid selection of specific treatments[62], such as imatinab for *Bcr-Abl*-positive chronic myeloid leukaemia.

The main developments in this field relate to pharmacogenomics – the tailoring of pharmacological treatment of disease or pre–disease states to possession of genetic variants that influence response[163; 164]. Proponents of this approach anticipate that developments will 'improve the chances of choosing the right drug for a patient by categorising patients into genetically definable classes that have similar drug effects'[63]. In addition to tailoring treatment, pharmacogenetics in the common disease context seeks to optimise treatment response, reduce side effects and contribute to appropriate scheduling and dosage of pharmacological treatment [2; 3; 4; 64; 65]. As in other areas of genetic epidemiology, pharmacogenetics has historically been characterised by persistent optimism in the face of failure to replicate initial claims of common variants being related to drug responsivity, which is likely to be at least partially due to poor study design and inadequate sample sizes[66]. One study, for example, reported an apparently robust difference in response to statin therapy; two variant forms of the HMG coenzyme A reductase (*HMGCR*) gene were associated with a 42 versus 33 mg/dl difference in total cholesterol[67]. Such a difference would be unlikely to influence clinical practice, however, because the reductions in low–density lipoprotein cholesterol in both groups would be expected to give substantial cardioprotection. Certainly, possession of these variants does not constitute statin 'responder' or 'non–responder' status, as suggested by commentators on this study[3]. Knowledge of *HMGCR* genotype seems incapable of influencing management decisions in any useful way, and this conclusion is strengthened by more recent studies that have failed to replicate the initial findings with respect to the *HMGCR* genetic variants and statin response[168;169].

Pharmacogenomics is clearly a rapidly developing field and further evidence needs to be gathered to evaluate whether genetic testing has both clinical benefit and is cost effective. Pragmatic randomised controlled trials should be the aim in this area, in which the outcomes and costs of drug treatment with and without information from genetic testing are assessed[3]. The SEARCH trial for abacavir hypersensitivity discussed above provides an exemplar of the sort of randomised controlled trials that are needed to in pharmacogenetic research.

Mendelian randomisation: strengthening causal inference in observational epidemiology

The basic aim of aetiological observational epidemiology is to identify modifiable causes of disease, and through this contribute to strategies for prevention. Thus observational studies have provided strong evidence that high circulating cholesterol levels and blood pressure increase the risk of coronary heart disease[68] – findings later confirmed in randomised controlled trials. The reputation of this enterprise has, however, received several setbacks in recent years, with observational studies apparently having identified robust associations, interpreted as probably or possibly causal, that, when tested in randomised controlled trials, have proved to be illusory[69; 70]. Hormone replacement therapy and coronary heart disease[71; 72], beta–carotene and lung cancer[73; 74], vitamin C and coronary heart disease[75; 76], dietary fibre and colon cancer[77], and vitamin E and coronary heart disease[78; 79] are examples of this. It is obvious that the candidate causes receiving the strongest support from observational and mechanistic studies will be the ones to be first evaluated in randomised controlled trials, and therefore it is probable that the myriad of associations reported from observational studies that have not been tested in controlled trials are less likely to be truly causal.

Why have observational studies and randomised controlled trials yielded different findings? The most plausible reason in the cases discussed above is confounding, as we summarise with respect to vitamin C and coronary heart disease in Figure 7.1. Despite attempts to adequately control for confounding, this has proved difficult when the exposure under study is related to a wide range of other factors influencing disease risk. In such situations appropriately designed genetic epidemiological studies can contribute to drawing robust inferences, using an approach that has come to be termed 'Mendelian randomisation' (Box 7.3).

The basic principle used in such studies is that if genetic variants either alter the level of, or mirror the biological effects of, a modifiable environmental exposure that itself alters disease risk, then these genetic variants should be related to disease risk to the extent predicted by their influence on exposure to the risk factor. Common genetic polymorphisms that have a well characterised biological function (or are markers for such variants) can therefore be used to study the effect of a suspected environmental exposure on disease risk[5; 10].

It may seem paradoxical to study genetic variants as proxies for environmental exposures rather than measure the exposures themselves. However, there are several crucial advantages of using functional genetic variants (or their markers) in this manner. Firstly, unlike environmental exposures, genetic variants are not

Figure 7.1: Comparisons between observational and randomised evidence of the effect of vitamin C on coronary heart disease risk

Studies included are the Heart Protection Study, the EPIC observational cohort study and the British Women's Heart & Health Study (BWHHS). Data are sequentially adjusted for potential confounders. Figures on the right are odd ratios with 95% confidence intervals. The better the adjustment for confounders, the closer the finding of the observational study (BWHHS) is to that of the randomised controlled trial (Heart Protection Study). Unfortunately, confounders can never be perfectly measured, and in many cases in observational studies there is residual confounding after adjustment for measured confounders. SEP, socioeconomic position.

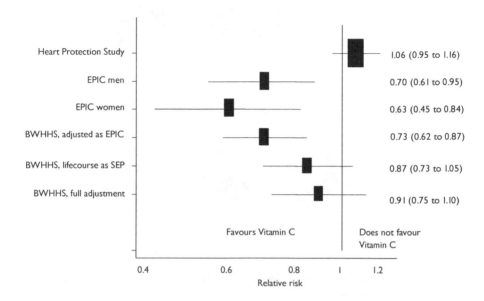

generally associated with the wide range of behavioural, social and physiological factors that, for example, confound the association between vitamin C and coronary heart disease (Box 7.2). Further, aside from the effects of population structure (see Chapter Four) such variants will not be associated with other genetic variants, excepting those with which they are in linkage disequilibrium. This latter assumption follows from the law of independent assortment (sometimes referred to as Mendel's second law); hence the term 'Mendelian randomisation'. We illustrate these powerful aspects of Mendelian randomisation in Box 7.3, showing the strong associations between a wide range of variables and blood C-reactive protein (CRP) levels, but no association of the same factors with genetic variants in the *CRP* gene. The only factor related to genotype is the expected, biological, influence of the genetic variant on CRP levels. This demonstration of the generally non-confounded nature of genetic variants was extended through a comprehensive analysis of 96 phenotypes and 23 genotypes, in which it was shown that there are no more conventionally significant associations between genotype and phenotype than would be expected by chance[170].

Secondly, inferences drawn from observational studies are subject to bias resulting from reverse causation. Disease processes may influence exposure levels; for

How the media often portray epidemiological studies

Observational epidemiology: confusing the public?

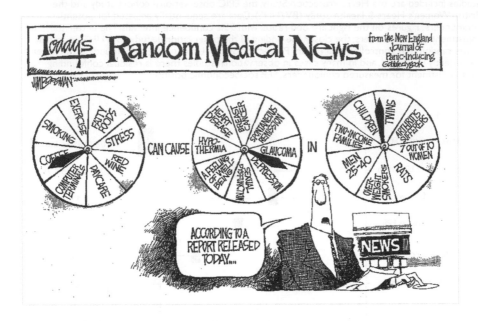

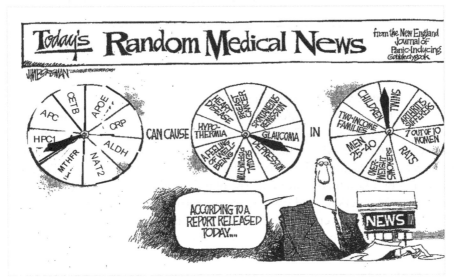

© Jim Borgman 2011

Box 7.3: Why 'Mendelian randomisation'?

Gregor Mendel (1822-1884) concluded from his hybridisation studies with pea plants that 'the behaviour of each pair of differentiating characteristics [such as shape of the seeds and colour of the seeds] in hybrid union is independent of the other differences between the two original plants'[135]. This formulation was actually the only regularity that Mendel referred to as a 'law' and in Carl Correns' 1900 paper (one of a trio appearing that year that are considered to represent the rediscovery of Mendel), he refers to this as 'Mendel's law'[136; 182]. Morgan[183] discusses independent assortment and refers to this process as being realised 'whenever two pairs of characters freely Mendelise.' Morgan's use of Mendel's surname as a verb did not catch on, but Morgan later christened this principle 'Mendel's second law'[184] and it has been known as this, or as the 'Law of Independent Assortment' since that time. The law suggests that the inheritance of one trait is independent of – that is, randomised with respect to – the inheritance of other traits. The analogy with a randomised controlled trial will clearly be most applicable to parent-offspring designs investigating the frequency with which one of two alleles from a heterozygous parent is transmitted to offspring with a particular disease[5]. However, at a population level, traits influenced by genetic variants are generally not associated with the social, behavioural and environmental factors that confound relationships observed in conventional epidemiological studies. Thus although the 'randomisation' is approximate and not absolute in genetic association studies, empirical observations suggest that it applies in most circumstances[170; 185; 186] (see Table 7.3).

The term 'Mendelian randomisation' itself was first introduced in a somewhat different context, in which the random assortment of genetic variants at conception is used to provide an unconfounded study design for estimating treatment effects for childhood malignancies[137; 138]. The term has recently become widely used with the meaning we ascribe to it in this chapter.

The notion that genetic variants can serve as an indicator of the action of environmentally modifiable exposures has been expressed in many contexts. For example, since the mid-1960s various investigators have pointed out that the autosomal dominant condition of lactase non-persistence is associated with reduced milk drinking. Associations of lactase non-persistence with osteoporosis, low bone mineral density or fracture risk thus provide evidence that milk drinking protects against these conditions[139; 140]. In a related vein, it was proposed in 1979 that as N-acetyltransferase pathways are involved in the detoxification of arylamine, a potential bladder carcinogen, the observation of increased bladder cancer risk among people with genetically determined slow acetylator phenotype provided evidence that arylamines are involved in the aetiology of the disease[141].

Since that time various commentators have pointed out that the associations of genetic variants of known function with disease outcomes provides evidence about aetiological factors[142–6]. However, these commentators have not emphasised the key strengths of Mendelian randomisation – the avoidance of confounding, of bias due to reverse causation or reporting tendency, and of the underestimation of risk associations due to variability in behaviours and phenotypes[187].

Some of these key concepts were present in Martijn Katan's 1986 *Lancet* letter, in which he suggested that genetic variants related to cholesterol level could be used to investigate whether the observed association between low cholesterol and increased cancer risk was real[80], and in a paper by Honkenen and colleagues in their understanding of how lactase persistence could better characterise the difficult-to-measure environmental exposure of calcium intake than could direct dietary reports[84]. Since 2000 there have been many reports using the term 'Mendelian randomisation' in the way it is used here[5; 12; 13; 14], and its use is becoming widespread. The fact that Mendelian randomisation is one of a family of techniques referred to as 'instrumental variable' approaches for obtaining robust causal inferences from observational data has also been recognised and developed[117; 161].

example ill people may start drinking less alcohol, or illness can influence measures of intermediate phenotypes such as cholesterol levels and fibrinogen. Martijn Katan's original proposition of what today is termed Mendelian randomisation[80] was that although the early stages of cancer could lower circulating levels of cholesterol (thus generating a misleading inverse association between cholesterol level and future risk of cancer mortality), germline genetic variants associated with cholesterol levels would not be altered by the development of cancer. Thus if there were a causal inverse association between cholesterol level and cancer risk, people carrying genotypes associated with lower cholesterol levels should have an increased risk of developing cancer.

Thirdly, many environmental exposures may be subject to reporting bias. For example, alcohol intake is often poorly reported, with a tendency for heavy drinkers to underestimate their intake[81; 82]. It is widely believed that moderate wine drinking, rather than other alcohol beverages, is cardioprotective. This may have introduced a reporting bias in case–control studies investigating this hypothesis as people with coronary disease under-reporting wine consumption, with reduced odds of coronary heart disease in moderate wine drinkers observed in some of the studies[83]. By contrast, in cohort studies, in which alcoholic drink preferences are measured before onset of disease, such a reporting tendency will not arise, perhaps explaining the more consistent findings of cardioprotective effects from all types of alcoholic drinks, irrespective of type in cohort studies[83]. A genetic variant related to exposure will not, of course, be altered by knowledge of disease status. Thus the strong association between the null variant of the aldehyde dehydrogenase 2 gene (*ALDH2*) and usual level of alcohol consumption (see later) would mean that *ALDH2* genotype can serve as a useful – unbiased and unconfounded – marker of usual alcohol consumption level before the development of disease[10].

Finally, a genetic variant will indicate long-term levels of exposure, and if the variant is taken as a proxy for such exposure, it will not suffer from the measurement error inherent in phenotypes that have high levels of variability. For example, groups defined by cholesterol-level-related genotype will, over a long period, experience the cholesterol difference seen between the groups. For individuals, blood cholesterol is variable over time, and the use of single measures of cholesterol will underestimate the true strength of association between cholesterol and, say, coronary heart disease. Indeed, use of the Mendelian randomisation approach predicts a strength of association that is in line with randomised controlled trial

Table 7.3a: The relationship between blood pressure, pulse pressure, hypertension and potential confounders according to concentration of C-reactive protein

	Means or proportions by quartiles of CRP (range) (mg/l)				
	1st quartile (0.16-0.85)	2nd quartile (0.86-1.71)	3rd quartile (1.72-3.88)	4th quartile (3.89-112.0)	p trend across categories
Hypertension (%)	45.8	49.7	57.5	60.0	< 0.001
BMI (kg/m²)	25.2	27.0	28.5	29.7	< 0.001
HDLc (mmol/l)	1.80	1.69	1.00	1.53	< 0.001
Lifecourse socioeconomic position score	4.08	4.37	4.46	4.75	< 0.001
Doctor diagnosis of diabetes (%)	3.5	2.8	4.1	8.4	< 0.001
Current smoker (%)	7.9	9.6	10.9	15.4	< 0.001
Physically inactive (%)	11.3	14.9	20.1	29.6	< 0.001
Moderate alcohol consumption (%)	22.2	19.6	18.8	14.0	< 0.001

Means or proportions of blood pressure, pulse pressure, hypertension and potential confounders are shown by quartiles of C-reactive protein concentration. n = 3,529[104]. BMI, body mass index; CRP, C-reactive protein; HDLc, high-density lipoprotein cholesterol.

Table 7.3b: Relationship between systolic blood pressure, hypertension and potential confounders and *CRP* 1059G/C genotype

	Genotype		
	GG	GC or CC	p
CRP (mg/l) (log scale)	1.81	1.39	< 0.001
Hypertension (%)	53.3	53.1	0.95
BMI (kg/m²)	27.5	27.8	0.29
HDLc (mmol/l)	1.67	1.65	0.38
Lifecourse socioeconomic position score	4.35	4.42	0.53
Doctor diagnosed diabetes (%)	4.7	4.5	0.80
Current smoker (%)	11.2	9.3	0.24
Physically inactive (%)	18.9	18.9	1.0
Moderate alcohol consumption (%)	18.6	19.8	0.56

Means or proportions of systolic blood pressure, hypertension and potential confounders are shown for each *CRP* 1059G/C genotype. From [104]. For CRP, geometric means and proportionate (%) change for a doubling of CRP are shown. BMI, body mass index; CRP, C-reactive protein; HDLc, high-density lipoprotein cholesterol.

findings of effects of cholesterol lowering, when the increasing benefits seen over the relatively short trial period are projected to the expectation for differences over a lifetime[10; 171].

Categories of Mendelian randomisation

There are several categories of inference that can be drawn from studies using the Mendelian randomisation paradigm. In the most direct forms genetic variants can be related to the probability or level of exposure ('exposure propensity') or to intermediate phenotypes believed to influence disease risk. Less direct evidence can come from genetic variant-disease associations that indicate that a particular biological pathway may be important, perhaps because the variants modify the effects of environmental exposures. As several examples of these categories have been given elsewhere[5; 10; 11; 172]; we will just briefly outline a few illustrative cases.

Exposure propensity

Osteoporosis may be related to habitual low calcium intake, but measuring propensity to exposure accurately is difficult. It has been suggested that assessing the association between calcium exposure and bone health can be done by comparing people with and without lactase persistence, as this may provide a better index of long-term low calcium intake[84]. Lactase persistence is an autosomal dominant condition, and polymorphism, A13910 T/C near the lactase phlorizin hydrolase gene, has been found. In post-menopausal women, the CC genotype is strongly associated with lactase non-persistence, low dietary intake of calcium from milk, a 10% lower bone mineral density at hip and spine and a greater risk of non-vertebral fractures[85] (Figure 7.2).

These relationships provide strong evidence that milk drinking improves bone health. This is particularly relevant because directly studying milk intake is potentially beset with problems of confounding, reverse causation (people with bone problems may be told to drink more milk) and measurement error. Indeed, in another field, claims of associations between milk drinking and reduced risk of coronary heart disease[86; 87] have been criticised for inadequately dealing with confounding and reverse causation[88].

A further example concerns the health consequences of alcohol use. Alcohol is oxidised to acetaldehyde, which in turn is oxidised by aldehyde dehydrogenases (ALDHs) to acetate. Approximately 50% of the Japanese population are heterozygotes or homozygotes for a null variant of *ALDH2* and peak blood acetaldehyde concentrations after alcohol challenge are 18 times and 5 times higher, respectively, among homozygous null variant and heterozygous individuals, compared with homozygous wild-type individuals[89]. This renders the consumption of alcohol unpleasant by inducing facial flushing, palpitations, drowsiness and other symptoms. As Figure 7.3a shows, there are considerable differences in alcohol consumption according to genotype[90]. The principles of

Figure 7.2a: Milk drinking and fracture risk according to lactose persistence genotype

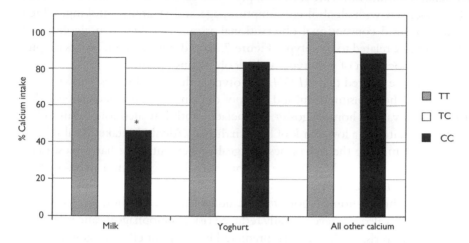

Notes: Individuals with genotype CC (dark bars) had lower calcium intake from milk (*p = 0.004) compared with TT (dashed bars) and TC (shaded bars) genotypes

Source: Obermayer Petsch *et al.* 2004

Figure 7.2b: Fracture incidence per 100 subjects in postmenopausal women according to *LCT* genotype

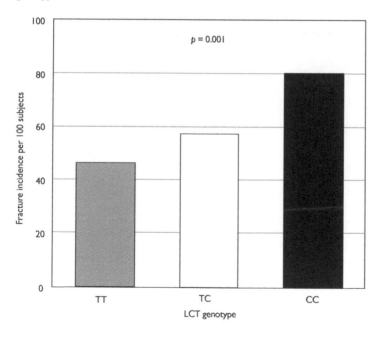

Mendelian randomisation are seen to apply – two factors that would be expected to be associated with alcohol consumption, age and cigarette smoking, which would confound conventional observational associations between alcohol and disease, are not related to genotype (Figure 7.3b and Figure 7.3c). This is despite the strong association of genotype with alcohol consumption.

It would be expected that *ALDH2* genotype influences diseases known to be related to alcohol consumption, and as proof of principle it has been shown that *ALDH2* null variant homozygosity – associated with low alcohol consumption – is indeed related to a lower risk of liver cirrhosis[91]. Alcohol intake has also been postulated to increase the risk of oesophageal cancer, but some have questioned the importance of its role[92]. Figure 7.4 presents findings from a meta-analysis of studies of *ALDH2* genotype and oesophageal cancer risk[93], clearly showing that people who are homozygous for the null variant, who therefore consume considerably less alcohol, have a greatly reduced risk of oesophageal cancer. Indeed, this reduction in risk is close to that predicted by the joint effect of genotype on alcohol consumption and the association of alcohol consumption on oesophageal cancer risk in a meta-analysis of such observational studies[94]. A similar situation is seen with respect to *ALDH2* genotype, alcohol intake and blood pressure levels; *ALDH2* genotype is associated with blood pressure to the extent predicted by the joint effects of genotype on alcohol intake and observational associations of

Figure 7.3: Relationship between alcohol intake, other characteristics and ALDH2 genotype

7.3a: Alcohol intake

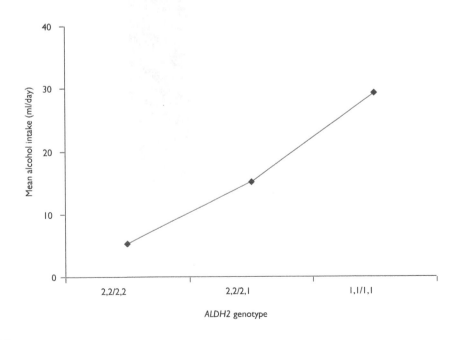

Figure 7.3b: Cigarette smoking (%)

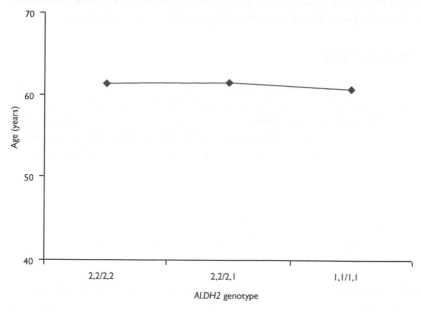

Figure 7.3c: Age (years)

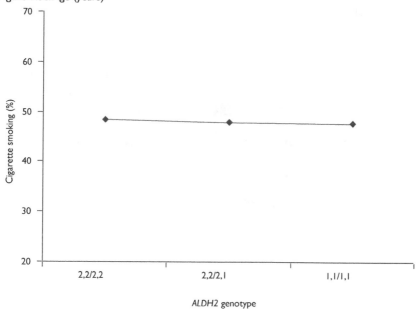

alcohol intake on blood pressure[173]. These associations provide strong evidence that alcohol intake does indeed causally influence blood pressure levels.

Intermediate phenotypes

Genetic variants can influence circulating biochemical factors such as cholesterol, homocysteine or fibrinogen levels. This provides a method for assessing causality in associations observed between these measures (intermediate phenotypes) and disease, and thus whether interventions to modify the intermediate phenotype could be expected to influence disease risk. Strong associations of CRP, an acute phase inflammatory marker, with hypertension, insulin resistance and coronary heart disease have been observed repeatedly[95-101], with the obvious inference that CRP is a cause of these conditions[102; 103]. A Mendelian randomisation study demonstrated that although serum CRP differences were highly predictive of blood pressure and hypertension, the CRP genetic variants – which predict sizeable

Figure 7.4: Risk of oesophageal cancer in individuals with the *ALDH2* 2,2 versus *ALDH2* 1,1 genotype

CI, confidence interval

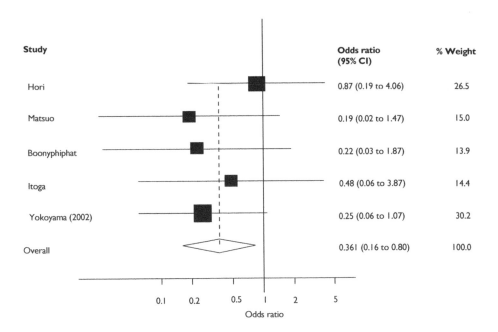

Study	Odds ratio (95% CI)	% Weight
Hori	0.87 (0.19 to 4.06)	26.5
Matsuo	0.19 (0.02 to 1.47)	15.0
Boonyphiphat	0.22 (0.03 to 1.87)	13.9
Itoga	0.48 (0.06 to 3.87)	14.4
Yokoyama (2002)	0.25 (0.06 to 1.07)	30.2
Overall	0.361 (0.16 to 0.80)	100.0

Source: [93]

serum CRP differences – were not associated with these same outcomes[104]. It is likely that these divergent findings are explained by complex confounding between serum CRP and outcomes (as shown in Table 7.3). Current evidence on this issue, suggests that CRP levels do not lead to elevated risk of hypertension, insulin resistance, diabetes or coronary heart disease[9; 105]. Similar findings have been reported for serum fibrinogen, variants in the beta fibrinogen gene and coronary heart disease[5-12; 174].

Identifying biological pathways to disease

The suggestion that taking aspirin reduces the risk of colon cancer originated from a case–control study exploring a large number of potential risk factors[106] and has been replicated in other studies[107]. Taking a Mendelian randomisation approach allows the important biological pathway to be identified, as aspirin has many effects. By examining variants in the gene coding for prostaglandin H synthase 2 (*PTGS2*), an enzyme involved in conversion of arachidonic acid to prostaglandin H_2 that is inhibited by aspirin[108], an association was found with reduced colon cancer risk. The investigators hypothesised that naturally occurring *PTGS2* variants might mimic long-term aspirin use. A larger study is required to confirm these exciting preliminary data. The data do, however, provide supportive evidence that aspirin (and other *PTGS2* inhibitors) protects against colon cancer, and that this protection is due to an inhibition of the conversion of arachidonic acid to prostaglandin. Positive findings have been reported from two small randomised trials of aspirin in high-risk patients, providing further evidence in support of a causal role for aspirin[109; 110]. Combining data from observational epidemiological studies, Mendelian randomisation designs and randomised controlled trials provides a powerful basis for causal inference.

Modifiers of environmental exposure

Sheep dip may be hazardous because of the organophosphates contained in it, but the vague symptoms farm workers attribute to exposure are not considered by some to be causal, but rather to be motivated by the prospect of secondary gain from compensation[111; 112]. Conducting trials would be unethical and valid observational studies impossible, as reporting bias would be likely to occur. Variants of the paraoxonase gene that produce different forms of the enzyme paraoxonase, with varying ability to detoxify organophosphates, can be used to indicate the effects of different levels of sheep dip exposure. If organophosphates in sheep dip truly cause ill health, then among people exposed to sheep dip, a higher proportion of those with symptoms would be expected to carry the genetic variants related to less efficient detoxification, and this is what has been found (Cherry *et al.* 2002). Given that it is unlikely that possession of the detoxification genotype is related to the tendency to report symptoms differentially, or to the desire for compensation, these findings provide evidence that sheep dip, and not compensation neurosis, is the cause of farm workers' symptoms. However, the lack of association of reporting tendency with genotype cannot be assumed and should be explicitly examined, and in this case the Mendelian randomisation approach would be formulated in terms of an expected gene–environment interaction (Box 7.4).

Intergenerational influences – methyl-tetrahydrofolate reductase polymorphisms and neural tube defects

Examining the effects of mother's genotype (independent of genotype of offspring) on the health outcomes of their offspring is a form of 'intergenerational' Mendelian randomisation, providing evidence on the role of intrauterine environment on the health of children. For example, periconceptual and early pregnancy folate deficiency is now known to be a cause of neural tube defects (NTDs), an effect confirmed by randomised controlled trial evidence[113; 114]. The methyl-tetrahydrofolate reductase (MTHFR) 677C/T polymorphism is associated with increased blood levels of homocysteine (equivalent to the result of lower levels of

---

Box 7.4: Mendelian randomisation and gene-environment interactions

Many of the inferences from Mendelian randomisation approaches come from main effects of genotypes (such as *ALDH2* or *CRP* variants and disease outcomes). This is advantageous, as relying on main effects avoids the issue of the greatly increased multiple statistical testing when interactions are looked for, the problem that exposure misclassification decreases ability to detect interaction and the scale dependency in the statistical conceptualisation of interactions[5; 13]. Some hypotheses would, however, need to be addressed through the expectation of interactions. For example, the role of paraoxanase variants in detecting causal effects of organophosphate-containing sheep dips would be best supported by finding that the paraoxanase variants are related to symptoms in those exposed to sheep dip but not in the unexposed. Similarly the role of environmental tobacco smoke in lung cancer aetiology would be supported by finding that detoxification variants are related to lung cancer risk in those exposed to environmental tobacco smoke but not in the unexposed[147], although current studies have not explicitly examined this[148]. In these situations, if there is exposure misclassification – for example if some of those reporting they were not exposed to sheep dip were exposed – the effect estimates for the genetic variants within exposures categories would be biased towards each other (and those in the supposedly unexposed group away from the null) and these formulations lose the strength of main-effect Mendelian randomisation studies as they are not protected from biased classification according to an environmental exposure. The interpretation of gene by environment interactions within a Mendelian randomisation framework is discussed at length elsewhere[162].

folate intake) and in a meta-analysis of case-control studies of NTDs, TT mothers had a twofold higher risk of having an infant with a NTD than CC mothers[115]. The relative risk of a neural tube defect associated with the TT genotype in the infant was less than that associated with the maternal genotype, and there was no effect of paternal genotype on offspring neural tube defect risk. This suggests that it is the intra-uterine environment – influenced by maternal TT genotype– rather than the genotype of offspring that increases the risk of NTD[5; 115].

Implications of Mendelian randomisation study findings

Establishing the causal influence of environmentally modifiable risk factors from Mendelian randomisation designs informs policies for improving population health through population-level interventions, *not* through genetic screening to identify those at high risk. For example, the implications of studies on maternal *MTHFR* genotype and offspring NTD risk is that population risk for NTDs can be reduced through increased folate intake periconceptually and in early pregnancy. It does not suggest that women should be screened for *MTHFR* genotype; women without the TT genotype but with low folate intake still carry a preventable risk of having babies with NTDs. Similarly, establishing the association between genetic variants (such as familial defective ApoB) associated with elevated cholesterol level and coronary heart disease risk strengthens causal evidence that elevated cholesterol is a modifiable risk factor for coronary heart disease across the whole population; thus, even though the population-attributable risk for coronary heart disease of this variant is small, it usefully informs public health approaches to improving population health. It is this aspect of the approach that illustrates its distinction from conventional risk identification and genetic screening uses of genetic epidemiology.

Limitations of Mendelian randomisation

Limitations of Mendelian randomisation have been discussed previously [5; 7; 8; 116; 117] (Box 7.5). A major limitation is common to all genetic association studies; the failure to establish reliable associations between genotype and intermediate phenotype, or between genotype and disease. This is probably largely related to the limited sample size of many current studies[118].

Although control of confounding is one of the advantages of Mendelian randomisation, it is possible that confounding could arise either through one genetic variant being in linkage disequilibrium with another functional variant as a result of population stratification, or through pleiotropy, the multiple function of genes. The issue of population stratification is discussed in Chapter Four. Linkage disequilibrium of one functional variant with another that influences the same disease outcome, but through another pathway, is of course also possible, but the short-range nature of linkage disequilibrium in most of the human genome may render this a relatively unusual phenomenon. Pleiotropy may be more problematic

Box 7.5: Limitations of Mendelian randomisation
- Failure to establish reliable associations between genotype and intermediate phenotype or between genotype and disease
- Confounding of associations between genotype, intermediate phenotype and disease through linkage disequilibrium or population stratification
- Pleiotropy and the multi-functionality of genes
- Canalisation and developmental stability
- Complexity of interpretations of associations between genotype, intermediate phenotype and disease
- Lack of suitable polymorphisms for studying modifiable exposures of interest

– it is increasingly evident that alternative splicing and related phenomena may lead to genes having multiple phenotypic consequences. One obvious strategy here is that potential confounders should be examined in relation to genotype (as we do in Table 7.3b, for example), rather than relying on the principle of Mendelian randomisation. However, this detracts from the particular power of Mendelian randomisation, as unmeasured confounders and measurement error limit the power of this approach. It may be possible to identify two separate genetic variants, which are not in linkage disequilibrium with each other but which both serve as proxies for the environmentally modifiable risk factor of interest. If both variants are related to the outcome of interest and point to the same underlying association then it becomes much less plausible that reintroduced confounding explains the association, because it would have to be acting in the same way for these two unlinked variants. This can be likened to randomised controlled trials of different blood-pressure-lowering agents, which work through different mechanisms and have different potential side effects, but which lower blood pressure to the same degree. If the different agents produce the same reductions in cardiovascular disease risk then it is unlikely that this is through agent-specific effects of the drug; rather it points to blood pressure lowering as being key. The use of multiple genetic variants working through different pathways has not been explicitly applied in Mendelian randomisation to date, but is an important potential development in the methodology. Indeed, the multiple genetic variants that have now been related to both cholesterol level and coronary heart disease risk constitute an informal demonstration of this multiple instrument approach.

Developmental compensation can occur. If a person has developed and grown from the intra-uterine period onwards within an environment in which one factor is perturbed by a particular genetic variant, they may be rendered resistant to its influence by permanent changes in tissue structure and function that counterbalance its effects – so called 'canalisation'[5; 119; 120; 121]. For example, it is possible that the effect of a difference in level of an intermediate phenotype (such as circulating cholesterol) that has been expressed from the period of intrauterine development onwards would have a different effect from that produced by modification of the intermediate phenotype in adulthood because of such developmental compensation. Little is known as to the actual importance of this, but 'knockout' animal preparations – with complete removal of the expression of particular genes from conception – have often produced phenotype changes that are considerably less severe than anticipated[122; 123; 124]. For genotypes that proxy for environmental exposures in postnatal life (such as *ALDH2* variants and alcohol consumption) or interact with postnatal exposures (such as paraoxanase variants and organophosphate metabolism), or when maternal genotypes are used to study intra–uterine influences, canalisation should not generally be an issue. In other cases, knowledge of when a gene is expressed, or whether gene-gene interactions might be expected (on the basis of knowledge of intermediate phenotype effects), can provide some insight into the probable role of canalisation in distorting interpretations from Mendelian randomisation designs.

The interpretation of findings from studies that appear to fall within the Mendelian randomisation remit can often be complex, as has been discussed elsewhere with respect to *MTHFR* and folate intake[10]. As a further example, consider the association of extracellular superoxide dismutase (EC-SOD) and coronary heart disease. EC-SOD is an extracellular scavenger of superoxide anions and thus genetic variants associated with higher circulating EC-SOD levels might be considered to mimic higher levels of antioxidants. However, findings are dramatically opposite to this – bearers of such variants have an increased risk of coronary heart disease[125]. The explanation of this apparent paradox may be that the higher circulating EC-SOD levels associated with the variant may arise from movement of EC-SOD from arterial walls: the in situ antioxidative properties of these arterial walls are weaker in individuals with the variant associated with higher circulating EC-SOD. The complexity of these interpretations – together with their sometimes speculative nature – detracts from the transparency that otherwise makes Mendelian randomisation attractive.

An obvious limitation of Mendelian randomisation is that it can examine only areas for which there are functional polymorphisms (or genetic markers linked to such functional polymorphisms) that are relevant to the modifiable exposure of interest. In the context of genetic association studies more generally, it has been pointed out that in many cases, even if a locus is involved in a disease-related metabolic process, there may be no suitable marker or functional polymorphism to allow study of this process[175]. The authors of this chapter have previously discussed the example of vitamin C in a Mendelian randomisation context[176], as a well known example of how observational epidemiology appears to have got the wrong answer relates to vitamin C and coronary heart disease[177]. The association between vitamin C and coronary heart disease could have been studied using the principles of Mendelian randomisation. Polymorphisms exist that are apparently related to lower circulating vitamin C levels – for example, the haptoglobin polymorphism[178; 179] – but in this case the effect on vitamin C is at some distance from the polymorphic protein and, as in the apolipoprotein E example, other phenotypic differences could have an influence on coronary heart disease risk that would distort the relationships of genotype, vitamin C levels and disease.

SLC23A1 – a gene encoding the vitamin C transporter SVCT1, which is involved in vitamin C transport by intestinal cells – would be an attractive candidate for Mendelian randomisation studies. However, by 2003 (the date of the example in our earlier paper) a search for variants had failed to find any common SNPs that could be used in such a way[180]. This was therefore used as an example of a situation in which suitable polymorphisms for studying the modifiable risk factor of interest – in this case vitamin C – could not be located. However, since the earlier paper was written, functional variation in *SLC23A1* has been identified that is related to circulating vitamin C levels (our unpublished work). This example is used not to suggest that the obstacle of locating relevant genetic variation for particular problems in observational epidemiology will always be overcome, but to point out that rapidly developing knowledge of human genomics will identify more variants that can serve as instruments for Mendelian randomisation studies.

Conclusion

It seems likely that fundamental gains in public health will eventually result from a steady growth in our understanding of the ways in which genes and environment act together to influence risk of complex disease[181]. A substantial part of this growth in knowledge and understanding may arise from the new methods to model causal pathways, such as the Mendelian randomisation strategy, but the correct interpretation of this concept is intimately tied up with a sound understanding of the underlying biology. It is important that biomedical and public health scientists use the investment in genetic epidemiology wisely and avoid overstating the pace at which returns can realistically be expected.

References
1. Bell J, Predicting disease using genomics. *Nature Review*, 2004; 429, 453-456.
2. Johnson JA, Pharmacogenetics: potential for individualised drug therapy through genetics. *Trends in Gentics*, 2003, 19, 660-666.
3. Haga SB, Burke W, Using Pharmocogenetics to Improve Drug Safety and Efficacy. *JAMA*, 2004; 291, 2869-2871.
4. Evans WE, Relling MV, Moving towards individualised medicine with pharmacogenomics. *Nature*, 2004; 429, 464-468.
5. Davey Smith G, Ebrahim S, 'Mendelian randomisation': can genetic epidemiology contribute to understanding environmental determinants of disease? *International Journal of Epidemiology*, 2003; 32, 1-22.
6. Davey Smith G, Harbord R, Ebrahim S, Fibrinogen, C-reactive protein and coronary heart disease: does Mendelian randomisation suggest the associations are non-causal? *Quarterly Journal of Medicine*, 2004; 97, 163-166.

7. Brennan P, Commentary: Mendelian randomisation and gene-environment interaction. *International Journal of Epidemiology*, 2004; 33, 17-21.

8. Tobin MD, Minelli C, Burton PR, Commentary: Development of Mendelian randomisation: from hypothesis test to 'Mendelian deconfounding'. *International Journal of Epidemiology*, 2004; 33, 21-25.

9. Keavney B, Commentary: Katan's remarkable foresight: genes and causality 18 years on. *International Journal of Epidemiology*, 2004; 33, 11-14.

10. Davey Smith G, Ebrahim S, Mendelian randomisation: prospects, potentials, and limitations. *International Journal of Epidemiology*, 2004; 33, 30-42.

11. Davey Smith G, Randomised by (your) god: unbiased effect estimates from an observational study design. *Journal of Epidemiology and Community Health*, 2006; 60,382-388.

12. Youngman LD, Keavney BD, Palmer A, *et al.*, Plasma fibrinogen and fibrinogen genotypes in 4685 cases of myocardial infarction and in 6002 controls: test of causality by "Mendelian randomisation". *Circulation*, 2000; 102, suppl II, 31-32.

13. Clayton D, McKeigue PM, Epidemiological methods for studying genes and environmental factors in complex diseases. *Lancet*, 2001; 358, 1356-60.

14. Fallon UB, Ben-Shlomo Y, Davey Smith G, (2001) *Homocysteine and coronary heart disease, Heart Online*, http://heart.bmjjournals.com/cgi/eletters/85/2/153

15. Caskey CT, DNA-Based Medicine: Prevention and Therapy. In: Kevles DJ, Hood L (eds.) *The Code of Codes: Scientific and Social Issues in the Human Genome Project*. London: Harvard University Press, 1993, 112-135.

16. Watson JD, A Personal View of the project. In: Kevles DJ, Hood L (eds.) *The Code of Codes: Scientific and Social Issues in the Human Genome Project*. London: Harvard University Press, 1993, 164-173.

17. Bell J, The new genetics in clinical practice. *British Medical Journal*, 1998; 31, 618-620.

18. Collins FS, Medical and Societal Consequences of the Human Genome Project. *New England Journal of Medicine*, 1999; 341, 28-37

19. Thakkinstian A, Han P, Smith W, *et al.*, Systematic review and meta-analysis of the association between complementary factor H Y402H polymorphisms and age-related macular degeneration. *Human Molecular Genetics*, 2006; 15, 2784-2790.

20. Grody WW, Molecular genetic risk screening. *Annual Review of Medicine*, 2003; 54, 473-90.

21. Genetic testing for cystic fibrosis, National Institutes of Health Consensus Development Conference Statement on genetic testing for cystic fibrosis. *Archives of Internal Medicine*, 1999; 159, 1529-1539.

22. Grody WW, Cutting GR, Klinger KW, *et al.*, Laboratory standards and guidelines for population-based cystic fibrosis carrier screening. *Genetic Medicine*, 2001; 3, 149-154.

23. American College of Obstetrics and Gynecology and American College of Medical Genetics. *Preconception and prenatal carrier screening for cystic fibrosis, clinical and laboratory guidelines, 2001.* Washington, DC: American College of Obstetrics and Gynecology publication, 2001.

24. Strom CM, Crossley B, Redman JB, *et al.*, Cystic fibrosis screening: Lessons learned from the first 320,000 patients. *Genetic Medicine,* 2004; 6, 136-140

25. Vastag B, Cystic fibrosis gene testing a challenge. *JAMA*, 2003; 289, 2923-2924.

26. Palomaki GE, Prenatal screening for cystic fibrosis: An early report card. *Genetic Medicine*, 2004; 6, 115-116.

27. Richards CS, Grody WW, Prenatal screening for cystic fibrosis: past, present and future. *Expert Review of Molecular Diagnostics*, 2004; 4, 49-62.

28. Gordon C, Walpole I, Zubrick SR, *et al.*, Population screening for cystic fibrosis: Knowledge and emotional consequences 18 months later. *American Journal of Medical Genetics*, 2003; 120A, 199-208.

29. Marteau TM, Dundas R, Axworthy D, Long-term cognitive and emotional impact of genetic testing for carriers of cystic fibrosis: The effects of test result and gender. *Health Psychology*, 1997; 16, 51-62.

30. Marteau TM, Michie S, Miedzybrodzka ZH, *et al.*, Incorrect recall of residual risk three years after carrier screening for cystic fibrosis: A comparison of two-step and couple screening. *American Journal of Obstetrics and Gynecology*, 1999; 181, 165-169.

31. Honnor M, Zubrick SR, Walpole I, *et al.*, Population screening for cystic fibrosis in Western Australia: Community response. *American Journal of Medical Genetics*, 2000; 93, 198-204.

32. Clausen H, Brandt NJ, Schwartz M, *et al.*, Psychological and social impact of carrier screening for cystic fibrosis among pregnant women – a pilot study. *Clinical Genetics*, 1996; 49, 200-205.

33. Eng CM, Schechter C, Robinowitz J, *et al.*, *JAMA,* 1997; 278, 1268-1272.

34. Eng CM, Desnick RJ, Experiences in molecular-based prenatal screening for Ashkenazi Jewish genetic diseases. Advances in Genetics, 2001; 44, 275-96.

35. Norio R, Finnish disease Heritage I: characteristics, causes, background. *Human Genetics*, 2003; 112, 441-456.

36. Pastinen T, Perola M, Ignatius J, *et al.,* Dissecting a population genome for targeted screening of disease mutations. *Human Molecular Genetics,* 2001; 10, 2961-2972.

37. Godard B, ten Kate L, Evers–Kiebooms G, *et al.,* Population genetic screening programmes: principles, techniques, practices, and policies. *European Journal of Human Genetics,* 2003; 11, Suppl 2, S49-87.

38. Feder JN, Gnirke A, Thomas W, *et al.,* A novel MHC class I–like gene is mutated in patients with hereditary haemochromatosis. Nature Genetics, 1996; 13, 399-408.

39. Byrnes V, Ryan E, Barrett S, *et al.,* Genetic hemochromatosis, a Celtic disease: is it now time for population screening? *Genetic Testing,* 2001; 5, 127-30.

40. Niederau C, Strohmeyer G, Strategies for early diagnosis of haemochromatosis. *European Journal of Gastroenterology and Hepatology,* 2002; 14, 217-21.

41. Witte DL, Crosby WH, Edwards CQ, *et al.,* Practice guideline development task force of the College of American Pathologists. Hereditary hemochromatosis. *Clinica Chimica Acta,* 1996; 245, 139-200

42. Beaudle*t al.,* Making genomic medicine a reality. *American Journal of Human Genetics,* 1999; 64, 1-13

43. Humphries SE, Ridker PM, Talmud PJ, Genetic testing for cardiovascular disease susceptibility: a useful clinical management tool or possible misinformation? *Arteriosclerosis, Thrombosis, and Vascular Biology,* 2004; 24, 628-36.

44. Ye Z, Liu EH, Higgins JP, *et al.,* Seven haemostatic gene polymorphisms in coronary disease: meta-analysis of 66,155 cases and 91,307 controls. *Lancet,* 2006; 367, 651-8.

45. Eby N, Chang-Claude J, Bishop DT, Familial risk and genetic susceptibility for breast cancer. *Cancer Causes Control,* 1994; 5, 458-70.

46. Antoniou A, Pharoah PD, Narod S, *et al.,* Average risks of breast and ovarian cancer associated with BRCA1 or BRCA2 mutations detected in case Series unselected for family history: a combined analysis of 22 studies. American Journal of Human Genetics, 2003; 72, 1117-30.

47. Griffith GL, Edwards RT, Gray J, *et al.,* Estimating the survival benefits gained from providing national cancer genetic services to women with a family history of breast cancer. *British Journal of Cancer,* 2004; 90, 1912-9.

48. Eccles DM, Hereditary cancer: guidelines in clinical practice. Breast and ovarian cancer genetics. *Annals of Oncology,* 2004; 15 Suppl 4, iv133-8.

49. McLeod HL, Krynetski EY, Relling MV, *et al.,* Genetic polymorphisms of *TPMT* and its clinical relevance for childhood acute lymphoblastic leukaemia. *Leukemia,* 2000; 14, 567-62

50. McCarthy TV, Quane KA, Lynch PJ, Ryanodine receptor mutations in malignant hyperthermia and central core disease. Human Mutation, 2000; 15, 410-7.

51. Vineis P, Schulte PA, Scientific and ethical aspects of genetic screening of workers for cancer risk: the case of the N–acetyltransferase phenotype. *Journal of Clinical Epidemiology,* 1995; 48, 189–97.

52. Haga SB, Khoury MJ, Burke W, Genomic profiling to promote a healthy lifestyle: not ready for prime time. *Nature Genetics,* 2003; 34, 347-50.

53. Klerk M, Verhoef P, Clarke R, *et al.,* MTHFR 677C T polymorphism and risk of coronary heart disease. A meta-analysis. *JAMA,* 2002; 288, 2023-2031.

54. Wald DS, Law M, Morris JK, Homocysteine and cardiovascular disease: evidence on causality from a meta-analysis. *British Medical Journal,* 2002; 325, 1202-1206

55. Scheuner MT, Genetic evaluation for coronary artery disease. *Genetic Medicine,* 2003; 5, 269-85.

56. Dekou V, Whincup P, Papacosta O, *et al.,* The effect of the C677T and A1298C polymorphisms in the methylenetetrahydrofolate reductase gene on homocysteine levels in elderly men and women from the British Regional Heart Study. *Atheroslcerosis,* 2001; 154, 659-666

57. Lewis S, Ebrahim S, Davey Smith G, Meta-analysis of MTHFR 677C->T polymorphism and coronary heart disease: does totality of evidence support causal role for homocysteine and preventive potential of folate? *British Medical Journal,* 2005; 331, 1053

58. Ebrahim S, Montaner D, Lawlor DA, Clustering of risk factors and social class in childhood and adulthood in British women's heart and health study: cross sectional analysis. *British Medical Journal,* 2004; 328, 861.

59. Khoury MJ, Yang Q, Gwinn M, *et al.,* An epidemiologic assessment of genomic profiling for measuring susceptibility to common diseases and targeting interventions. *Genetic Medicine,* 2004; 6, 38–47.

60. Yoon PW, Scheuner MT, Peterson-Oehlke KL, *et al.,* Can family history be used as a tool for public health and preventive medicine? *Genetic Medicine,* 2002; 4, 304–10.

61. Guttmacher AE, Collins FS, Carmona RH, The family history--more important than ever. *New England Journal of Medicine,* 2004; 351, 2333-6.

62. Workman P, The opportunities and challenges of personalised genome-based molecular therapies for cancer: targets, technologies, and molecular chaperones. *Cancer Chemotherapy & Pharmacology,* 2003; 52, Suppl 1, S45-56

63. Kalow W, Pharmacogenetics and personalised medicine. *Fundamental & Clinical Pharmacology,* 2002; 16,5, 337–42.

64. Oscarson M, Pharmacogenetics of drug metabolising enzymes: importance for personalised medicine. *Clinical Chemistry & Laboratory Medicine,* 2003; 41, 4, 573-80.

65. Goldstein DB, Tate SK, Sisodiya SM, Pharmacogenetics goes genomic. *Nature Reviews Genetics,* 2003; 4, 937-947.

66. Kajinami K, Takekoshi N, Brousseau ME, *et al.,* Pharmacogenetics of HMG–CoA reductase inhibitors: exploring the potential for genotype-based individualisation of coronary heart disease management. *Atherosclerosis,* 2004; 177, 219-234.

67. Chasman DI, Posada D, Subrahmanyan L, *et al.,* Pharmacogenetic study of statin therapy and cholesterol reduction. *JAMA,* 2004; 291, 2821-2827.

68. Stamler J, *Lectures on Preventive Cardiology.* New York: Grune & Stratton, 1967.

69. Taubes G, Epidemiology faces its limits. *Science,* 1995; 269, 164-69.

70. Davey Smith G, Reflections on the limitations to epidemiology. *Journal of Clinical Epidemiology,* 2001; 54, 325-331.

71. Stampfer MJ, Colditz GA, Estrogen replacement therapy and coronary heart disease: a quantitative assessment of the epidemiologic evidence. *Preventive Medicine,* 1991; 20,47-63. (reprinted *International Journal of Epidemiology,* 2004; 33, 445-453).

72. Petitti D, Commentary: Hormone replacement therapy and coronary heart disease: four lessons. *International Journal of Epidemiology,* 2004; 33, 461 – 463.

73. Willett WC, Vitamin A and lung cancer. *Nutrition Review,* 1990; 48, 201-11.

74. Alpha-Tocopherol, Beta Carotene Cancer Prevention Study Group. The effect of vitamin E and beta carotene on the incidence of lung cancer and other cancers in male smokers. *New England Journal of Medicine,* 1994; 330, 1029-35.

75. Khaw K-T, Bingham S, Welch A, *et al.,* Relation between plasma ascorbic acid and mortality in men and women in EPIC-Norfolk prospective study: a prospective population study. *Lancet,* 2001; 357, 657-63.

76. Heart Protection Study Collaborative Group, MRC/BHF heart protection study of antioxidant vitamin supplementation in 20,536 high-risk individuals: a randomised placebo-controlled trial. *Lancet,* 2002; 360, 23-33.

77. Lawlor DA, Ness AR, Commentary: The rough world of nutritional epidemiology: Does dietary fibre prevent large bowel cancer? *International Journal of Epidemiology,* 2003; 32, 239-243.

78. Rimm EB, Stampfer MJ, Ascherio A, *et al.,* Vitamin E consumption and the risk of coronary heart disease in men. *New England Journal of Medicine,* 1993; 328, 1450-1456.

79. Shekelle PG, Morton SC, Jungvig LK, *et al.,* Effect of supplemental vitamin E for the prevention and treatment of cardiovascular disease. *Journal of General Internal Medicine,* 2004; 19, 380-389.

80. Katan MB, Apolipoprotein E isoforms, serum cholesterol, and cancer. *Lancet,* 1986; I, 507-508. (reprinted *International Journal of Epidemiology,* 2004; 349).

81. Buchsbaum DG, Welsh J, Buchanan RG, *et al.,* Screening for drinking problems by patient self-report. Even 'safe' levels may indicate a problem. *Archives of Internal Medicine,* 1995; 155, 104-8.

82. Fuller RK, Lee KK, Gordis E, Validity of self-report in alcoholism research: results of a Veterans Administration Cooperative Study. *Alcoholism: Clinical & Experimental Research,* 1998; 12, 201-5.

83. Rimm EB, Klatsky A, Grobbee D, *et al.,* Review of moderate alcohol consumption and reduced risk of coronary heart disease: is the effect due to beer, wine, or spirits? *British Medical Journal,* 1996; 312: 731-736.

84. Honkanen R, Pulkkinen P, Järvinen R, *et al.,* Does lactose intolerance predispose to low bone density? A population-based study of perimenopausal Finnish women. *Bone,* 1996; 19, 23-28.

85. Obermayer-Pietsch BM, Bonelli CM, Walter DE, *et al.,* Genetic Predisposition for Adult Lactose Intolerance and Relation to Diet, Bone Density, and Bone Fractures. *Journal of Bone and Mineral Research,* 2004; 19, 42-7.

86. Elwood PC, Milk, coronary disease and mortality. *Journal of Epidemiology and Community Health,* 2001; 55, 375.

87. Ness AR, Davey Smith G, Hart C, Milk, coronary heart disease and mortality. *Journal of Epidemiology and Community Health,* 2001; 55, 379-382.

88. Shaper AG, Wannamethee G, Walker M. Milk, butter and heart disease. *British Medical Journal,* 1991; 302, 785-6.

89. Enomoto N, Takase S, Yasuhara M, *et al.,* Acetaldehyde metabolism in different aldehyde dehydrogenase-2 genotypes. *Alcoholism: Clinical Experimental Research,* 1991; 15, 141-4.

90. Takagi S, Iwai N, Yamauchi R, *et al.,* Aldehyde dehydrogenase 2 gene is a risk factor for myocardial infarction in Japanese men. *Hypertension Research,* 2002; 25, 677-681.

91. Chao Y-C, Liou S-R, Chung Y-Y, *et al.,* Polymorphism of alcohol and aldehyde dehydrogenase genes and alcoholic cirrhosis in Chinese patients. *Journal of Hepatology,* 1994; 19, 360-366

92. Memik F, Alcohol and esophageal cancer, is there an exaggerated accusation? *Hepatogastroenterology,* 2003; 54, 1953-5

93. Lewis S, Davey Smith G, Alcohol, ALDH2 and esophageal cancer: A meta-analysis which illustrates the potentials and limitations of a Mendelian randomisation approach. *Cancer Epidemiology, Biomarkers and Prevention,* 2005; 14, 1967-1971.

94. Gutjahr E, Gmel G, Rehm J, Relation between average alcohol consumption and disease: an overview. *European Addiction Research,* 2001; 7, 117-27.

95. Danesh J, Wheeler JG, Hirschfield GM, *et al.,* C-reactive protein and other circulating markers of inflammation in the prediction of coronary heart disease. *New England Journal of Medicine,* 2004; 350, 1387-97

96. Wu T, Dorn JP, Donahue RP, *et al.*, Associations of serum C-reactive protein with fasting insulin, glucose, and glycosylated hemoglobin: the Third National Health and Nutrition Examination Survey, 1988-1994. *American Journal of Epidemiology*, 2002; 155, 65-71

97. Pradhan AD, Manson JE, Rifai N, *et al.*, C-reactive protein, interleukin 6, and risk of developing type 2 diabetes mellitus. *JAMA*, 2001; 286, 327-34

98. Han TS, Sattar N, Williams K, *et al.*, Prospective study of C-reactive protein in relation to the development of diabetes and metabolic syndrome in the Mexico City Diabetes Study. *Diabetes Care*, 2002; 25, 2016-21

99. Freeman DJ, Donahue RP, Sempos CT, *et al.*, Associations of serum C-reactive protein with fasting insulin, glucose, and glycosylated hemoglobin: the Third National Health and Nutrition Examination Survey, 1988-1994. *American Journal of Epidemiology*, 2002; 155, 65-71

100. Sesso D, Buring JE, Rifai N, *et al.*, C-reactive protein and the risk of developing hypertension. *JAMA*, 2003; 290, 2945-2951

101. Hirschfield GM, Pepys MB, C-reactive protein and cardiovascular disease: new insights from an old molecule. *Quarterly Journal of Medicine*, 2003; 9, 793-807

102. Ridker PM, Cannon CP, Morrow D, *et al.*, C-reactive protein levels and outcomes after statin therapy. *New England Journal of Medicine*, 2005; 352, 20-8

103. Sjöholm A, Nyström T, Endothelial inflammation in insulin resistance. *Lancet*, 2005; 365, 610-2

104. Davey Smith G, Lawlor D, Harbord R, *et al.*, Association of C-reactive protein with blood pressure and hypertension: lifecourse confounding and Mendelian randomisation tests of causality. *Arteriosclerosis, Thrombosis, and Vascular Biology*, 2005; 25: 1051–1056.

105. Zee RYL, Ridker PM, Polymorphism in the human C-reactive protein (CRP) gene, plasma concentrations of CRP, and the risk of future arterial thrombosis. *Atherosclerosis*, 2002; 162, 217-9

106. Kune GA, Kune S, Watson LF, Colorectal cancer risk, chronic illnesses, operations and medications: case control results from the Melbourne Colorectal Cancer Study. *Cancer Research*, 1988; 48, 4399-4404.

107. Sandler RS, Galanko JC, Murray SC, *et al.*, Aspirin and nonsteroidal anti-inflammatory gents and risk for colorectal adenomas. *Gastroenterology*, 1998; 114, 441-447.

108. Lin HJ, Lakkides KM, Keku TO, *et al.*, Prostaglandin H Synthase 2 variant (Val511Ala) in African Americans may reduce the risk for colorectal neoplasia. *Cancer Epidemiology, Biomarkers and Prevention*, 2002; 11, 1305-1315.

109. Sandler RS, Halabi S, Baron JA, *et al.*, A randomised trial of aspirin to prevent colorectal adenomas in patients with previous colorectal cancer. *New England Journal of Medicine*, 2003; 348, 883–890

110. Baron JA, Cole BF, Sandler RS, *et al.*, A randomised trial of aspirin to prevent colorectal adenomas. *New England Journal of Medicine*, 2003; 348: 891–899

111. BBC Online (1999) *Report raises sheep dip health fears*, http://news.bbc.co.uk/1/hi/health/383003.stm

112. BBC Online (1999) *Jury out on sheep dip*, http://news.bbc.co.uk/1/hi/health/537549.stm

113. MRC Vitamin Study Research Group. Prevention of neural tube defects: Results of the Medical Research Council vitamin study. *Lancet*, 1991; 338, 131–37.

114. Czeizel AE, Dudás I, Prevention of the first occurrence of neural–tube defects by periconceptional vitamin supplementation. *New England Journal of Medicine*, 1992; 327, 1832–5.

115. Botto LD, Yang Q, 5, 10-Methylenetetrahydrofolate reductase gene variants and congenital anomalies: a HuGE Review. *American Journal of Epidemiology*, 2000; 151, 862–77.

116. Little J, Khoury MJ, Mendelian randomisation: a new spin or real progress? *Lancet*, 2003; 362, 930–931.

117. Thomas DC, Conti DV. Commentary on the concept of "Mendelian Randomisation". *International Journal of Epidemiology*, 2004; 33, 17–21.

118. Colhoun H, McKeigue PM, Davey Smith G, Problems of reporting genetic associations with complex outcomes. *Lancet*, 2003; 361, 865–72.

119. Waddington CH, Canalisation of development and the inheritance of acquired characteristics. *Nature*, 1942; 150, 563–5.

120. Wilkins AS, Canalisation: a molecular genetic perspective. *BioEssays*, 1997; 19, 257–262.

121. Hartman JL, Garvik B, Hartwell L, Principles for the buffering of genetic variation. *Science*, 2001; 291, 1001–4

122. Langenbach R, Morham SG, Tiano HF, *et al.*, Prostaglandin synthase gene disruption in mice reduces arachidonic acid-induced inflammation and indomethacin-induced gastric ulceration. *Cell*, 1995; 83, 483–492

123. De Witt D, Smith WL, Yes, but do they still get headaches? *Cell*, 1995; 83, 345–8

124. Godecke A, Schrader J, Adaptive mechanisms of the cardiovascular system in transgenic mice--lessons from eNOS and myoglobin knockout mice. *Basic Research in Cardiology*, 2000; 95, 492–8

125. Juul K, Tybjaerg-Hansen A, Marklund S, *et al.*, Genetically reduced antioxidative protection and increased ischaemic heart disease risk: The Copenhagen city heart study. *Circulation*, 2004, 109, 59–65.

126. Colhoun HM, McKeigue PM, Davey Smith G, Problems of reporting genetic associations with complex outcomes. *Lancet*, 2003; 361, 865–72

127. Ioannidis JP, Trikalinos TA, Ntzani EE, *et al.,* Genetic associations in large versus small studies: an empirical assessment. *Lancet*, 2003; 361, 567-71

128. Khachaturian AS, Corcoran CD, Mayer LS, *et al.,* Cache County Study Investigators. Apolipoprotein E epsilon4 count affects age at onset of Alzheimer disease, but not lifetime susceptibility: The Cache County Study. *Archives of General Psychiatry*, 2004; 61, 518-24.

129. Qiu C, Kivipelto M, Aguero-Torres H, *et al.,* Risk and protective effects of the APOE gene towards Alzheimer's disease in the Kungsholmen project: variation by age and sex. *Journal of Neurology, Neurosurgery and Psychiatry*, 2004; 75, 828-33

130. Severi G, Giles GG, Southey MC, *et al.,* ELAC2/HPC2 polymorphisms, prostate-specific antigen levels, and prostate cancer. *Journal of the National Cancer Institute*, 2003; 95, 818-24.

131. Frayling IM, Beck NE, Ilyas M, *et al.,* The APC variants I1307K and E1317Q are associated with colorectal tumors, but not always with a family history. *Proceedings for the National Academy of Sciences USA*, 1998; 95, 10722-7.

132. Hahnloser D, Petersen GM, Rabe K, *et al.,* Boardman L. *et al.* The APC E1317Q variant in adenomatous polyps and colorectal cancers. *Cancer Epidemiology, Biomarkers & Prevention*, 2003; 12, 1023-8

133. Statement on use of apolipoprotein E testing for Alzheimer disease. American College of Medical Genetics/American Society of Human Genetics Working Group on ApoE and Alzheimer disease. *JAMA*, 1995; 274: 1627 - 1629.

134. The UK National Screening Committee's Criteria for appraising the viability, effectiveness and appropriateness of a screening programme. www.doh.gov.uk/nsc/library/lib_ind.htm.

135. Mendel G, Experiments in plant hybridisation (1866). www.mendelweb. org/archive/Mendel.Experiments.txt

136. Correns CG, Mendel's Regel über das Verhalten der Nachkommenschaft der Bastarde. *Berichte der Deutschen Botanischen Gesellschaft*, 1900; 8, 158-68. English translation, G. Mendel's law concerning the behaviour of progeny of varietal hybrids, *Stern and Sherwood*, 1966; 119-32.

137. Gray R, Wheatley K, How to avoid bias when comparing bone marrow transplantation with chemotherapy. *Bone Marrow Transplantation*, 1991; 7, suppl 3, 9-12

138. Wheatley K, Gray R, Commentary: Mendelian randomisation – an update on its use to evaluate allogeneic stem cell transplantation in leukaemia. *International Journal of Epidemiology*, 2004; 33, 15-17.

139. Birge SJ, Keutmann HT, Cuatrecasas P, *et al.,* Osteoporosis, intestinal lactase deficiency and low dietary calcium intake. *New England Journal of Medicine*, 1967; 276, 445-448.

140. Newcomer AD, Hodgson SF, Douglas MD, *et al.*, Lactase deficiency: Prevalence in Osteoporosis. *Annals of Internal Medicine*, 1978; 89, 218-220.

141. Lower GM, Nilsson T, Nelson CE, *et al.*, N-acetylransferase phenotype and risk in urinary bladder cancer: approaches in molecular epidemiology. *Environmental Health Perspectives*, 1979; 29, 71-9.

142. McGrath J, Hypothesis: is low prenatal vitamin D a risk-modifying factor for schizophrenia? *Schizophrenia Research*, 1999; 40, 173-7

143. Ames BN, Cancer prevention and diet: Help from single nucleotide polymorphisms. *Proceedings for the National Academy of Sciences USA*, 1999; 96, 12216-18.

144. Rothman N, Wacholder S, Caporaso NE, *et al.*, The use of common genetic polymorphisms to enhance the epidemiologic study of environmental carcinogens. *Biochimica et Biophysica Acta*, 2001; 1471, C1-C10.

145. Brennan P, Gene environment interaction and aetiology of cancer: what does it mean and how can we measure it? *Carcinogenesis*, 2002; 23, 3, 381-387.

146. Kelada SN, Eaton DL, Wang SS, *et al.*, The role of genetic polymorphisms in environmental health. *Environmental Health Perspectives*, 2003; 111, 1055-64.

147. Davey Smith G, Effect of passive smoking on health. *British Medical Journal*, 2003; 326, 1048-1049.

148. Vineis P, Airoldi L, Veglia P, *et al.*, Environmental tobacco smoke and risk of respiratory cancer and chronic obstructive pulmonary disease in former smokers and never smokers in the EPIC prospective study. *British Medical Journal*, 2005; 330, 277.

149. Thompson A, Di Angelantonio E, Sarwar N, *et al.*, Association of cholesteryl ester transfer protein genotypes with CETP mass and activity, lipid levels, and coronary risk. JAMA, 2008; 299, 2777-88.

150. Willer CJ, Sanna S, Jackson AU, *et al.*, Newly identified loci that influence lipid concentrations and risk of coronary artery disease. *Nature Genetics*, 2008; 40, 161-9.

151. Zhou W, Liu G, Thurston SW, et al., Genetic polymorphisms in N-acetyltransferase-2 and microsomal expoxide hydrolase, cumulative cigarette smoking, and lung cancer. *Cancer Epidemiology, Biomarkers and Prevention*, 2002; 11, 15-21.

152. McKay JD, Hashibe M, Hung RJ, *et al.*, Sequence variants of NAT1 and NAT2 and other xenometabolic genes and risk of lung and aerodigestive tract cancers in Central Europe. *Cancer Epidemiology, Biomarkers and Prevention*, 2008; 17, 141-7.

153. Harold D, Abraham R, Hollingworth P, et al., Gonome-wide association study identifies variants at CLU and PICALM associated with Alzheimer's disease. *Nature Genetics*, 2009; 41, 1088-93.

154. Meigs JB, Shrader P, Sullivan LM, *et al.*, Genotype score in addition to common risk factors for prediction of type 2 diabetes. *New England Journal of Medicine*, 2008; 359, 2208-19.

155. Lyssenko V, Jonsson A, Almgren P, *et al.*, Clinical risk factors, DNA variants, and the development of type 2 diabetes. *New England Journal of Medicine*, 2008; 359, 2220-32.

156. SEARCH collaborative group: Link E, Parish S, Armitage J, *et al.*, SLCO1B1 variants and statin-induced myopathy – a genome-wide study. *New England Journal of Medicine*, 2008; 359, 789-99.

157. Daly AK, Donaldson PT, Bhatnagar P, *et al.*, for the DILIGEN study and International SAE Consortium, HLA-B★5701 genotype is a major determinant of drug-induced liver injury due to flucloxacillin. Nature Genetics, 2009; 41, 816-21.

158. Freathy R, Ring SM, Shields B, *et al.*, A common genetic variant in the 15q24 nicotinic acetylcholine receptor gene cluster (CHRNA5-CHRNA3-CHRNB4) is associated with a reduced ability of women to quit smoking in pregnancy. *Human Molecular Genetics*, 2009; 18, 2922-7.

159. Le Marchand L, Derby KS, Murphy SE, *et al.*, Smokers with the *CHRNA* lung cancer – associated variants are exposed to higher levels of nicotine equivalents and a carcinogenic tobacco-specific nitrosamine. *Cancer Research*, 2008; 68, 9137-40.

160. Wadman M, Gene-testing firms face legal battle. *Nature*, 2008; 453, 1148-9.

161. Lawlor DA, Harbord RM, Sterne JA, *et al.,* Mendelian randomization: using genes as instruments for making causal inferences in epidemiology. *Statistical Medicine*, 2008; 27, 1133-63.

162. Davey Smith G, Mendelian randomization for strengthening causal inference in observational studies: application to gene by environment interaction. *Perspectives on Psychological Science* 2010; 5, 527-45.

163. Zhang W, Ratain MJ, Dolan ME, The HapMap resource is providing new insights into ourselves and its application to pharmacogenomics. *Bioinformatics and Biology Insights*, 2008; 2, 15-23.

164. Davis RL, Khoury MJ, A public health approach to pharmacogenomics and gene-based diagnostic tests. *Pharmacogenomics*, 2006; 7, 331-7.

165. Lindgren CM, McCarthy MI, Mechanisms of disease: genetic insights into the etiology of type 2 diabetes and obesity. *Nature Clinical Practice Endocrinology and Metabolism,* 2008; 4, 156-63.

166. Thorgeirsson TE, Geller F, Sulem P, *et al.,* A variant associated with nicotine dependence, lung cancer and peripheral arterial disease. *Nature*, 2008; 452, 638-42.

167. Hung RJ, McKay JD, Gaborieau V, *et al.*, A susceptibility locus for lung cancer maps to nicotinic acetylcholine receptor subunit genes on 15q25. *Nature*, 2008; 452, 633-7.

168. Thompson JF, Man M, Johnson KJ, *et al.*, An association study of 43 SNPs in 16 candidate genes with atorvastatin response. *Pharmacogenomics Journal*, 2005; 5, 352-8.

169. Polisecki E, Muallem H, Maeda N, *et al.*, Genetic variation at the LDL receptor and HMG-CoA reductase gene loci, lipid levels, statin response, and cardiovascular disease incidence in PROSPER. *Atherosclerosis*, 2008; 200, 109-114.

170. Davey-Smith G, Lawlor DA, Harbord R, *et al.*, Clustered environments and randomized genes: a fundamental distinction between conventional and genetic epidemiology. *PLoS Medicine*, 2007; 4, e352.

171. Davey-Smith G, Timpson NJ, Ebrahim S, Strengthening causal inference in cardiovascular epidemiology through mendelian randomization. *Annals of Medicine*, 2008; 40, 7, 524-41.

172. Lawlor DA, Harbord RM, Sterne JA, *et al.*, Mendelian randomization: using genes as instruments for making causal inferences in epidemiology. *Stat Med* 2008; 27:1133-63.

173. Chen L, Davey Smith G, Harbord RM, *et al.*, Alcohol intake and blood pressure: a systematic review implementing a Mendelian randomization approach. *PLoS Medicine*, 2008; 5, e52.

174. Keavney B, Danesh J, Parish S, *et al.*, Fibrinogen and coronary heart disease: test of causality by 'Mendelian randomization'. *International Journal of Epidemiology*, 2006; 35, 935-43.

175. Weiss KM, Terwilliger JD, How many diseases does it take to map a gene with SNPs? *Nature Genetics*, 2000; 26, 151-7.

176. Davey Smith G, Ebrahim S, 'Mendelian randomization': can genetic epidemiology contribute to understanding environmental determinants of disease? *International Journal of Epidemiology*, 2003; 32, 1-22.

177. Dagenais GR, Marchioli R, Yusuf S, *et al.*, Beta-carotene, vitamin C, and vitamin E and cardiovascular diseases. *Current Cardiology Reports*, 2000; 2, 293-9.

178 Delanghe J, Langlois M, Duprez D, *et al.*, Haptoglobin polymorphism and peripheral arterial occlusive disease. *Atherosclerosis*, 1999; 145, 287-92.

179. Langlois MR, Delanghe JR, De Buyzere ML, *et al.*, Effect of haptoglobin on the metabolism of vitamin C. *American Journal of Clinical Nutrition*, 1997; 66, 606-10.

180. Erichsen HC, Eck P, Levine M, *et al.*, Characterization of the genomic structure of the human vitamin C transporter SVCT1 (SLC23A2). *Journal of Nutrition*, 2001; 131, 2623-7.

181. Palmer LJ, The New Epidemiology: putting the pieces together in complex disease aetiology. *International Journal of Epidemiology*, 2004; 33, 925-8.

182. Olby RC, *Origins of Mendelism*. London: Constable; 1966.

183. Morgan TH, *Heredity and sex*. New York: Columbia University Press; 1913.

184. Morgan TH, *Physical basis of heredity*. New York: Columbia University Press; 1918.

185. Davey Smith G, Lawlor DA, Harbord R, *et al.*, Association of C-reactive protein with blood pressure and hypertension: life course confounding and mendelian randomization tests of causality. *Arteriosclerosis, Thrombosis and Vascular Biology,* 2005; 25, 1051-6.

186. Bhatti P, Sigurdson AJ, Wang SS, *et al.*, Genetic variation and willingness to participate in epidemiologic research: data from three studies. *Cancer Epidemiology, Biomarkers and Prevention,* 2005; 14, 2449-53.

187. Smith GD, Ebrahim S, Mendelian randomization: prospects, potentials, and limitations. *International Journal of Epidemiology,* 2004; 33, 30-42.

Glossary

Words that are themselves defined in the glossary appear in **bold italics**.

Additive

An additive **allele** contributes one additional unit of quantity to the **base** level of the **phenotype** in a linear fashion. In **polygenic quantitative traits** such as height, the total effect of each additive allele on the phenotype is assumed to be small but equal to the effect of any additive allele at any other **locus**.

Allele

If the DNA sequence at a given **locus** (often a gene or a marker) varies between different **chromosomes** in the population, each different version can be called an allele. If there are two alleles at a given locus, the allele that is less common in the population can be designated the minor allele.

Amino acid

The organic building blocks that make up a protein or polypeptide.

Association study (genetic)

An investigation of the statistical association of an **allele** at a specific **locus** with a **phenotypic trait**.

Autosomal

Pertaining to the 22 non-sex **chromosomes** (in humans).

Base

See **nucleotide** and **base pairs**.

Base pairs (bp)

A measure of physical distance along a **chromosome**. When quantifying the length of a molecule of double stranded DNA, one enumerates the number of nucleotide **bases** along one strand. This is equivalent to counting the number of paired bases (A-T, C-G, G-C or T-A) along the two strands together.

Candidate gene

A gene that can be reasonably posited to be involved in the genesis of a **phenotypic trait** or disease on the grounds of biological plausibility.

Case

An individual in which the disease of interest is present.

Case–control study

Case–control studies are used to identify factors that may contribute to a medical condition by comparing people who have that condition (the '**cases**') with people who do not have the condition but are otherwise similar (the 'controls').

Centimorgan (cM)

A unit measuring *recombination* frequency used to infer genetic distance along a *chromosome*. One cM equals a 1% chance of recombination between two *loci* in a single generation. The unit is named after Thomas Hunt Morgan. The number of *base pairs* contained in a region of length 1.0 cM varies with gender, from place to place across the *genome* and by the mapping function used.

Chromosome, chromosomal

The human *genome* is broken up into 46 segments called chromosomes. There are 22 pairs of *autosomes* (numbered 1-22) and one pair of sex chromosomes (X,X in a female and X,Y in a male). The two chromosomes in a *homologous* pair, for example the two copies of chromosome 14, each have the same basic structure, including the same sequence of genes in the same places along the their length. However, they can vary in the precise sequence of the double stranded DNA at various positions along their length. One homologous chromosome in each pair is derived from an individual's mother and one from their father.

Co-dominance

A gene whose *alleles* do not exhibit dominance/recessiveness effects. Instead, the *heterozygous* individual expresses both *phenotypes*. The classic example of co-dominance is the ABO blood group system. The gene for blood types has three alleles: A, B and i. i causes O type and is *recessive* to both A and B. The A and B alleles are co-dominant with each other. When a person has both an A and a B allele, the person has type AB blood.

Codon

A *nucleotide* triplet that specifies a particular *amino acid* or indicates that protein *translation* should finish. For example, the *mRNA* triplet UAC codes for the amino acid tyrosine, as does UAU (exemplifying *redundancy in the genetic code*), and UAA is a stop codon: it indicates 'stop translation'.

Cohort study

A research design in which participants are selected on the basis of the presence or absence of a given *exposure* and then studied for a given period to establish disease *outcome* in each exposure group. Cohort studies may be either prospective or retrospective.

Common SNP

See *single nucleotide polymorphism*.

Complex disease

A disease that involves multiple genetic and environmental factors and that does not exhibit a classic Mendelian pattern of inheritance.

Confounder

An additional and often latent factor that might be responsible for an observed relationship between *exposure* and *outcome*. Confounding variables are associated with the exposure in question, and are independently associated with disease risk. By definition, a confounding variable is thus associated with both the probable cause and the outcome. The confounder may not be on the direct causal pathway between the explanatory variable and the outcome of interest. For instance, being male does not always lead to smoking tobacco, and smoking tobacco does not always lead to cancer. Therefore, in any study that tries to elucidate the relation between being male and cancer should take smoking into account as a possible confounder.

Crossover

At chiasma during the latter stages of meiotic cell division, crossover marks the point at which the process of breakage and reunion allows the physical exchange of genomic material between *homologous chromosome* arms. This forms the basis of a *recombination* event.

cSNP

Coding SNP. See *non-synonymous SNP*.

Diploid

Human somatic cells are diploid. They contain all 23 *chromosome* pairs: one copy of both members of each *homologous* pair (for example, two versions of chromosome 14). The full diploid human *chromosome* complement can be expressed as 46,XX in a female and 46,XY in a male.

Diplotype

An individual's *genotype* at multiple *loci* regardless of *haplotype* assignment.

Dominance

An *allele* that masks the effects of another allele at the same *locus* is said to be dominant.

Epistasis

The interaction between genes. Epistasis takes place when the action of one gene is modified by one or several other genes, which are sometimes called modifier genes.

Exon

A segment of a gene that is represented in mature/spliced RNA product. Individual exons typically include protein-coding sequences.

Exposure

A factor or situation of potential aetiological contribution to a given *trait* or disease to which an individual is exposed.

Familial

Aggregation of a *trait* in families of genetically related individuals.

Genetic heterogeneity

A characteristic of *complex diseases* whereby similar *phenotypes* can result from different *allelic* combinations.

Genetic marker

A variable DNA sequence that has a non-variable component that is sufficiently 'unique' to localise it to a single genomic *locus* and a variable component that is sufficiently heterogeneous to identify differences between individuals and between *homologous chromosomes* in an individual. Genetic markers play a pivotal role in gene mapping. Sequence variations at genetic markers do not usually cause direct coding changes in proteins.

Genome

The total genetic information carried by an individual or species.

Genotype

The genetic constitution of an individual at a particular *locus*, in other words the combination of *alleles* present at one locus. Usually expressed as two alleles in human genetics (such as AB), as humans have a *diploid chromosomal* complement.

Haploid

Gametes (sperm and ova) are haploid. They contain only one member of each *homologous chromosomal* pair (for example, only one version of chromosome 14).

All ova have chromosomal complement 23,X and all sperm have either 23,X or 23,Y. When sperm and ovum fuse to form a zygote, the *diploid* chromosomal complement is restored.

Haplotype

A series of *alleles* at *linked loci* along a single *chromosome*.

Heritability

The proportion of total *phenotypic* variance of a *quantitative trait* attributable to genetic factors. Broad sense heritability (h^2_B) estimates the proportion of total phenotypic variance attributable to all genetic factors, whereas narrow sense heritability (h^2_N) estimates the proportion of total phenotypic variance attributable to *additive* genetic factors.

Homologous chromosome pairs

See *chromosome*.

Homozygous

If the two *alleles* at a particular *locus* on a pair of *homologous chromosomes* are the same, the individual is said to be homozygous at that locus. If they are different the subject is *heterozygous*.

Heterozygous

See *homozygous*.

Incidence

A measure of the rate of occurrence of a disease over a specified period of time. Refers to the number of new *cases* (numerator) of a disease arising during a specified period in a defined population at risk (denominator).

Intron

Non-coding DNA that separates neighbouring *exons* in a gene.

Linkage

The situation in which two *syntenic loci* are inherited together. More specifically, two loci are said to be linked if they are close enough to each other on a *chromosome* such that *recombination* during meiosis is uncommon enough for their co-segregation to be detectable within families. Linkage analysis relies on statistical methods and seeks to estimate the recombination fraction (θ) between two or more loci in identifiable meiotic events.

Linkage disequilibrium (LD)

The increased frequency of *haplotypes* within a population due to co-inheritance of linked *alleles*. Any departure from the theoretical state of linkage equilibrium. Linkage disequilibrium leads to the statistical correlation between two *loci*.

Linked loci

Two *loci* that lie close enough together on a single *chromosome* that an *allele* at one locus has a tendency to be transmitted with the corresponding allele at the other locus (with the allele on the same chromosome) at gamete formation. Linked marker loci can be referred to as *linked markers* and marker loci that are not linked can be called *unlinked markers*.

Linked markers

See *linked loci*.

Locus (plural loci)

A locus is a unique *chromosomal* location defining the position of an individual gene or DNA sequence. In genetic *linkage* studies, the term can also be used to refer to a region involving one or more genes, perhaps including non-coding parts of the DNA.

Marker

See *genetic marker* and *linked loci*.

Messenger RNA (mRNA)

RNA transcribed from genes in nuclear DNA undergoes a series of post-transcriptional processing steps. The resultant mature mRNA is used as the template for the *translation* process that results in synthesis of a protein.

Microsatellite

Microsatellites consist of multiple repeats of a short sequence (typically 2-8 *base pairs*) such as 'CACACA...'. The *alleles* of a microsatellite are differentiated by the number of repeats they involve (for example, 'CA_{12}' denotes 12 CA repeats in a row).

Minor allele

See *allele*.

Most telomeric marker

See *telomere*.

mRNA

See *messenger RNA*.

Mutation

Novel DNA variants arise through mutation, which means a sequence change. A mutation can reflect anything from a single change at a *nucleotide* to a large scale *chromosomal* restructuring. A mutation in the germline (that is, in sperm or ova or in the cells that produce them) can be passed on to subsequent generations and can therefore cause heritable disease. Somatic mutations occur in non-germline cells; although they can cause serious disease (for example, some cancers), they cannot be inherited by offspring.

Non-synonymous SNPs

A *SNP* that alters the DNA sequence in a coding region in such a manner that a *codon* is changed so that it codes for an alternative *amino acid*, or changes from coding for an amino acid to specifying a stop *translation* signal, or vice versa. *Synonymous SNPs* alter the DNA sequence but do not change the protein coding sequence as interpreted at translation. This occurs because of *redundancy in the genetic code*: several different *codons* can specify the same amino acid. Non-synonymous SNPs can also be called coding SNPs or *cSNPs*.

Nucleotides

The organic building blocks that make up DNA and RNA. Composed of a ribose sugar, a purine or pyrimidine *base* and a phosphate group and taken as one functional unit in the framework of DNA.

Odds ratio (OR)

The ratio of the odds of a dichotomous *outcome* (such as being affected by a disease) among *exposed* individuals relative to that among unexposed individuals.

Oligogenic

Mode of inheritance involving several genes. Unlike strictly polygenic inheritance, oligogenic inheritance does not preclude major gene effects. See *polygenic*.

Outcome

The disease status of an individual after *exposure* to a particular factor.

Penetrance

The proportion of individuals carrying an *allele* who will express the *phenotype* associated with that allele; the probability of observing the phenotype given the specific *genotype*. The situation of less than 100% concordance between genotype and expected phenotype is referred to as reduced or incomplete penetrance.

Phase

The *haplotypic* configuration of *linked loci*. The *diplotype* U_1U_2–V_1V_2 is consistent with two possible phases: (i) U_1–V_1 on one *chromosome* and U_2–V_2 on the other; or (ii) U_1–V_2 on one chromosome and U_2–V_1 on the other. If a child receives U_1–V_1 on a paternally derived chromosome from a father with *diplotype* U_1U_2–V_1V_2 it either implies that the father was in phase (i) and no *recombination* has occurred or he was in phase (ii) and there has been a recombination.

Phenotype

In this book, we use the term phenotype interchangeably with the term *trait* to refer to a measurable characteristic of an individual, that is not itself a *genotype*.

Polygenic

The determination of a *trait* by multiple *loci*, each having a small *additive* effect.

Polymorphism

Genetic variation at a designated *locus* that occurs at an appreciable frequency in a given population. By definition, a locus that is polymorphic has at least two alternative *alleles*. Unfortunately, although its general meaning is uncontroversial, it also has several alternative definitions of a more specific nature – none of which is universally accepted. One important definition of this type is 'the existence of two or more genetic variants (alleles, [other] sequence variants, *chromosomal* structure variants) at significant frequencies in the population'[22]. But the term 'significant' in this definition is itself undefined. When the term polymorphism is used in this book, it will either be as one component of the term *single nucleotide polymorphism (SNP)* or else it will refer in general terms to a locus at which genetic variation is observed to occur. Unless otherwise made clear in the text, its usage will carry no implication about the type of variation that is observed, nor how common that variability may be.

Population stratification

The presence of a systematic difference in *allele* frequencies between subpopulations in a population, possibly due to different ancestry. Population stratification is also referred to as population structure. Population stratification can be a problem for *association studies*, such as *case-control studies*, in which a spurious association between an allele and disease status could be due to systematic differences in allele frequencies between *cases* and controls (that is, to underlying population structure).

Prevalence

Measure of disease frequency. Refers to the total number of *cases* (numerator) of the disease present in a population (denominator) at a given point in time.

Proband

The individual (usually affected) through whom a pedigree is ascertained.

Quantitative trait

A *trait* exhibiting continuous variation, such as height or weight. These traits are generally referred to as quantitative because they are studied using the quantitative tools of statistical analysis. Quantitative traits are generally thought to be affected by many genetic and environmental factors.

Recessive

An *allele* whose effect on *phenotypic* expression is 'masked' by that of another, *dominant* allele. In Mendelian genetics, recessive traits are expressed only in a *homozygote* for the recessive gene.

Recombination

The exchange of genetic material between two **homologous chromosomes** during meiosis, resulting in new genetic variation. In humans recombination occurs by crossing over during meiosis – the breaking down of one maternal and one paternal chromosome, the exchange of corresponding sections of DNA, and the rejoining of the chromosomes.

Redundancy in the genetic code

See **codon**.

Relative risk (RR)

Measure of disease-**exposure** relationship. Estimates the magnitude of an association between exposure and disease and indicates the likelihood of disease in exposed individuals compared with those who are not exposed. RR is the **incidence** of disease in the exposed group over the corresponding incidence in the non-exposed group. In a **case-control study**, RR is usually estimated using the **odds ratio**.

Replication

The biological process by which a molecule of double stranded DNA is copied to form two new, but identical, molecules of double stranded DNA.

Single nucleotide polymorphism (SNP)

A DNA variant in a single **nucleotide** (for example, the nucleotide present at a given position may be either T or G). A **common SNP** may be defined as a **locus** at which two SNP **alleles** are present, both at a frequency of ≥ 1%[97]. It has been estimated that, across the human **genome** as a whole, there are approximately 10 million common SNPs[97].

Synonymous SNPs

See **non-synonymous SNPs**.

Syntenic

On the same **chromosome**.

Telomere

Specialist structures at the tips of a **chromosome**. The term **most telomeric marker** (see Chapter Two) refers to the **marker** among a series of markers that is closest to the tip of the chromosome.

Trait

See **phenotype**.

Transcription

The synthesis of RNA on a DNA template.

Translation

The process whereby mature **messenger RNA** is decoded to specify the synthesis of proteins.

Index

Printed and bound by CPI Group (UK) Ltd, Croydon, CR0 4YY

27/10/2024

14580561-0001